Dedication

To the members of the human family who seek to know and learn of the correct diet for humans; and who are in pursuit of optimum health and longevity. This book is a testimony of the Guidance that can achieve those outcomes: How To Eat To Live, Volumes 1 & 2, written by the Honorable Elijah Muhammad. I advise everyone to read and follow the Divine Dietary Guidance given in those books.

Special Thanks

All Praise and Honor Belongs to Almighty Allah (God), Who Came in the Person of Master Fard Muhammad, the Great Mahdi, for Giving Humanity Divine Guides in the Persons of the Honorable Elijah Muhammad and the Honorable Minister Louis Farrakhan.

Special thanks to my beloved family: wife, Marcia; and children, Kevin, Jr., and Krystina for their great love and support. Also, thanking my wife for editing this work; my son for creating the graphics; and my daughter for persisting that I finish this book. I thank my God-filled mother, Helen Owens, for keeping me grounded in Almighty God; and my twin brother, Julian Muhammad, for his generosity and love.

I thank Bro. Jabril Muhammad (Phoenix, AZ), who twenty years ago, inspired me to delve deeper into the Life Giving Teachings of the Honorable Elijah Muhammad through an ever-increasing understanding of the Divine and Extraordinary Value of the Honorable Minister Louis Farrakhan. I also thank Sis. Judy Muhammad (Washington, D.C.), Sis. Linda Muhammad (Phoenix, Az), and Bro. Robert Muhammad (Wilmington, DE).

Special thanks to the Believers in Wilmington, Delaware; and all those wonderful souls who helped to make this work possible.

Nuts Are Not Good for Humans

Biological Consequences of Consumption

TechDoc, Incorporated
Newark, Delaware

Nuts Are Not Good for Humans: Biological Consequences of Consumption

Published in the United States by:
TechDoc, Incorporated
7 Waltham Street
Newark, Delaware 19713
www.etechpublish.com

Printed in the United States of America.

Main entry under title:
Nuts Are Not Good for Humans: Biological Consequences of Consumption

A TechDoc, Incorporated book
Bibliography: p.148, graphics

Library of Congress Card No. 00-100776
ISBN: 0-9658864-2-5

Cover designed by Studio A Productions, Wilmington, Delaware

Kevin A. Muhammad's website: *http://www.kamuhammad.net*

Table of Contents

Preface

For the past 20 years, I have benefited from the Divine and revolutionary dietary guidance given to humanity by Almighty God through the Honorable Elijah Muhammad. It has also been during these years that dietary issues have been pushed to the forefront of American and world concerns. Albeit, the Dietary Guidance given by the Honorable Elijah Muhammad predates, by some 50 years, the futile attempts of mainstream health institutions to offer appropriate dietary guidance. The futility of these efforts is evident in the epidemics of chronic and infectious diseases.

Many of these attempts have been unsuccessful because the motive out of which they sprung forth was to gain profit rather than to offer dietary guidance with the sole purpose of improving public health. The market is saturated with bogus health studies that tout certain foods or ingredients as miraculous substances. This has created a dietetic arena that is extremely confusing and contradictory. The danger associated with this debacle is that people are often injured.

I am among many who have become fed up with the mess that currently exist in the medical and dietetic communities. However, unlike many others, I have been afforded dietary guidance that has kept me out of harms way. The dietary guidance given by the Honorable Elijah Muhammad in the books, How To Eat To Live (volumes 1 and 2), has not left one stone unturned in addressing the foods that are both fit and unfit for human consumption. Those who follow this guidance have not had to wonder about this or that food being good to eat. Nor have our dietary position been compromised, in the least, by bogus health studies. We have long been taught that health is a commercial industry, and that following the sinister schemes of industry will only place us in an early grave.

According to the dietary law contained in the books, How To Eat To Live, nuts are among the foods that are unfit for human consumption. In fact, nuts are second only to swine flesh in the level of injury they cause when consumed. Nuts render a tremendous impact to human health. So, after witnessing the onslaught of nut-promotion studies over the past five years, I am obligated to combat this false dietary guidance.

This book, *Nuts Are Not Good for Humans,* is written to share with the public some of the dietary guidance contained in the books, How To Eat To Live. It also exposes the false dietary guidance rendered by so-called nutritionists and health institutions by presenting biochemical and biological research about nuts. This research, emphatically, proves that nuts are unfit for humans, and that nut-promoting studies are bogus and should not have been circulated through the media.

My hope is that people will have an opportunity to avoid the pitfalls created by false dietary advice, and gain greater health and longevity by following dietary guidance that has withstood the test of time—How To Eat To Live.

Introduction

Surveys show that people are aware of the impact of food on health and well-being.[1] They have learned this through their own eating habits. For example, many people have followed traditional dietary regimens that have made poor health a custom among their particular populations. Some of these traditional dishes feature high-fat, processed foods, which ensures that each generation confronts heart disease and other ailments associated with the consistent consumption of such foods.

According to epidemiological studies, poor diets are the primary cause of early mortality in the United States,[2] and as such, are associated with 6 of the 10 leading chronic diseases.[3] Chronic diseases prematurely claim the lives of millions each year, while causing massive suffering to millions of others. The price tag of this health burden is tremendous, driving national health expenditures to nearly a trillion dollars each year.[4]

Millions of people have also been injured after following nutritional advice from nutritional and medical practitioners, and government institutions. For example, for nearly 20 years the federal government has issued dietary recommendations, yet the overall health of the general population has worsened. This has made federally-sanctioned dietary advice suspect, and some organizations have opposed this advice. The recent release of the *2000 Dietary Guidelines for Americans* (Guidelines) is an example of this, as it was muddled with controversy.[5]

The Guidelines, which have been issued every five years for the past twenty years, sets dietary standards that influence the eating habits of Americans. Because of the impact that the Guidelines have on the eating behaviors of Americans, various health and public interest groups insisted that their positions be included in the document. This created a controversy that was unprecedented since the Guidelines were established.

In one instance, several organizations called for a de-emphasis on dairy products as a major dietary recommendation. They charged the dairy industry with wielding power over the direction of the Guidelines. They stood on research that alleged that milk and other dairy products are linked to heart disease, and therefore, should not be recommended for consumption.

In another instance, some groups called for a greater promotion of alcohol because several health studies had purported alcohol to contain health-promoting properties. Previous editions of the Guidelines merely advised people to consume alcohol in moderation. The groups, however, wanted alcohol to be given definitive consumption parameters.

These and other positions led to a significant overhaul of the 2000 Guidelines. When we consider these facts, confusing and contradictory dietary advice—professional, traditional, or otherwise—have caused the plague of diet-related chronic diseases. Extreme differences of opinion among health institutions about dietary issues have exacerbated the problem. So, despite the increased knowledge of agriculture, food technology, and medicine during the past 40 years, diet-related chronic diseases have remained epidemic. And, as we enter the 21st century, medical researchers expect this epidemic to worsen.[6]

The effort to reduce the current chronic disease epidemic, and stave off its imminent intensification, has lead to a re-emergence of nutritional and dietary recommendations. The market is now flooded with dietary advice—books, television programs, and other forms of medium. Many people and institutions are claiming to know the proper diet for humans. Most of this advice recommends the consumption of natural foods, such as beans, nuts, and other vegetation. The thought that vegetation is healthier for humans than meat is not a grand revelation.

This advice is acceptable because those who seek better health tend to gravitate toward diets that contain vegetables, fruits, and grains. Adhering to this advice appears to be a good start, but much remains desired, as chronic disease has continued to climb in spite of the promotion and increased consumption of natural foods. Such a situation appears paradoxical; however, many people have failed to ask a most important question: *Is a food good for health just because it's natural?*

Many assume that natural foods are good for human consumption. Generally, they are correct, but does this mean that all vegetables are safe to eat? *If all vegetables are not safe, then what are these vegetables? Why are they unhealthy? Can they be proven unhealthy?* The answers to these questions are critical, and represent a progressive step in the quest to secure appropriate dietary guidelines.

In the broadest sense, people know that all vegetation is not suitable to eat. At best, we learn of this through ailments that are brought about by the consumption of certain vegetables. When confronted with these discomforts, we resolve that the food did not "agree" with our digestive systems. After such experiences, people usually refrain from eating those foods. And, although a food that causes discomfort to one person may not do the same to another person, there are foods that cause harm to large segments of the population. Nuts, and certain beans and vegetables fall into this category. For example, beans are infamous for causing flatulence, and nuts are synonymous with allergic reactions.

In the food industry, however, the prevailing idea is that all vegetation is suitable to eat. The grocery stores are filled with the same foods eaten by other creatures, despite the fact that there are obvious anatomical differences between humans and other animals. Because there is no distinction among foods, humans eat the same foods as birds, cattle, and insects. Foods that are fit for these other creatures are usually unfit for humans.

Unfortunately, medical, health-related, and higher education institutions are the chief proponents of dietary advice that promote the consumption of foods that are unfit for humans. These entities craft so-called health studies to justify human consumption of poisonous animal foods. They are contributors, unknowingly or knowingly, to the chronic disease epidemic.

Among the most dangerous dietary advice currently rendered by these institutions is the recommendation to eat nuts. Not only are nuts being promoted as nutritious foods, but also as food with health promoting properties—eating them, purportedly, improves one's health. This nonsense is pervasively promoted in the media via published reports from notable institutions, such as Harvard and Penn State universities. As a result, nuts are being catapulted to greater prominence in the human food chain. This is an act that is sure to do greater harm than good. *Why*?

According to the Honorable Elijah Muhammad, nuts are unfit for humans and consuming them deals a tremendous blow to the human lifespan. He states that every time we eat nuts, five years are shaved from our life spans. Either this is exaggerative or it can be proven. Research into the biochemical constituents of nuts have confirmed them unfit for our consumption. Nuts contain potent poisons.

The problem is that the dietary advice of most, if not all, nutritionists is not based upon biochemical and biological analyses. Either they are unaware of this information, or simply choose to follow assumptions that have never been proven. There is greater proof that nuts are harmful than there is that they are beneficial.

The extraordinary negative impact that nuts render against human life deserves our attention. The thought that a mere serving of nuts erases five years from our lifespan implies that the results of their consumption are connected to leading chronic diseases. Such diseases include cancer, heart disease, and diabetes—the leading causes of early mortality. Thyroid disease, depression, osteoporosis and menopause are also linked to nut consumption.

The following chapters will show why nuts are not good for human consumption, and in doing so, describe the biological consequences associated with their consumption. Chapter 1 gives an overview of the use of nuts in human nutrition. Chapter 2 reviews the health studies that have promoted the consumption of nuts, while Chapter 3 challenges the validity of nut-promoting health studies.

Chapter 4 compares the human and avian (bird) digestive systems, thus showing the importance of anatomical differences when determining the foods that best serve humans. Chapter 5 describes the poisons contained in nuts and shows the potential biological impact that result when humans ingest these toxins. In Chapter 6, the association between nut consumption and chronic disease is described.

Chapters 7 and 8 describe the impact that nut poisons render against the human pancreas and thyroid gland, respectively. Chapter 9 describes the diseases that are associated with thyroid malfunction, and sheds greater light on the detriments of nut consumption.

Chapter 10 shows the mineral deficiencies that result from nut consumption, while Chapter 11 documents the contribution of nuts to the enormous allergy epidemic. Chapter 12 describes the pharmaceutical industry's success as evidence of the rise in diseases that result from poor dietary habits. Chapter 13 discusses the need to establish food distinctions in the human food chain.

CHAPTER

1

Nuts In Human Nutrition

Nuts have been a mainstay in the human diet for thousands of years and continue as a part of many diets throughout the world. The term "nuts" generally describes the shell-encased seeds of nonleguminous trees, but leguminous shell-encased seeds, such as peanuts, are also referred to as nuts. Nuts consumed as whole foods include coconuts, peanuts, almonds, walnuts, hazelnuts, pecans, cashew nuts, and pistachio nuts. These nuts are also used in many processed foods.

Although there are notable differences among nuts, there are some generalities with respect to their purported nutritional values. For example, most nuts contain approximately 500 or more calories (kcal) per 100-gram portions due to their high fat content; and thus, are generally viewed as fattening foods. Nuts contain only one-quarter to one-third as much carbohydrate as grains and legumes. They are also considered good sources of B-complex vitamins, and minerals.

The production of nuts in the United States represents only a small fraction of the world production, except in the case of almonds, where the United States contributes almost one-fourth of the world's production. Table 1 describes the world's most common nut crops.

The most important nut crops in the United States are almonds, coconuts, peanuts, pecans, and walnuts. With the exception of coconuts, the others have been the subjects of nutritional studies that promote their consumption. The following sections provide a brief overview of these nuts.

Almond

The almond is considered a member of the peach family. It is a native of Central Asia, but is now popular in the Mediterranean. Almonds have traditionally been a highly valued part of the diet of Mediterranean peoples. California is the major producer, followed by Spain, Portugal, and Italy.

Pecan

The pecan is the only major tree nut that grows naturally in North America and because of this, it is one of the most valuable North America nut species. The name "pecan" is a Native American word of Algonquin origin that was used to describe "all nuts requiring a stone to crack." It originated in central and eastern North America. Pecans were favored because they were accessible from waterways, and easier to unshell than other North American nut species.

Walnuts

Walnuts grew wild over a great portion of Europe and Asia, predating recorded history by thousands of years. The exact place and date of its origin is undetermined, but most authorities believe that the walnut first came from ancient Persia. Passed along in trade from Persia, walnuts became a popular food to the ancient peoples of Italy, Spain, Greece, India, China and Japan.

Walnuts were first introduced to California in the 1700's by the Spanish padres. It wasn't until the 1860's, however, that the industry was launched. Today, California produces most of the walnuts grown commercially in the United States.

Approximately 1.1 million tons of walnuts are harvested every year, and of that, about 20% is traded to countries. Production of walnuts has increased by nearly 40% in the last 20 years.

Peanut

The peanut, agriculturally, is a legume, although it is generally placed in the same category as tree nuts. It has been speculated that the peanut originated from semi arid areas of Brazil. The ancestors of the present Arawak Indian people domesticated it approximately 5,000 years ago. It was introduced to the United States from Africa. India, tropical Africa, and China are the leading peanut producing countries.

The peanut is noted for its high protein content. Peanuts and peanut butter contain 27-30% protein, which is increased in oil-free meals and flours to 50-55% protein. Whole peanuts contain about 50 grams of fats and 16 grams of carbohydrates per a 100-gram serving. About half the fat content is monounsaturated fat; a third is polyunsaturated; and a fifth is saturated.

In the United States, peanuts are a premiere crop, accounting for approximately 70% of the country's nut production. The peanut also ranks fourth after soybean, cottonseed and sunflower seed as an oilseed crop; and is fifth among vegetable oils produced.

It is important to note that the per capita consumption of peanuts in the United States is the highest in the world. The U.S. is the only country that consumes most of its peanut crop as whole-nut products. Approximately 2.4 billion pounds of peanuts are produced in the United States each year, and half of the nation's peanut crop is processed into peanut butter.[7]

Approximately 25-30% of the annual peanut production is roasted for consumption as whole-nut snacks, sweets, confections and baked goods. The remainder is crushed to produce oil and meal. The meal is used as animal feed or is processed into edible-grade, high-protein flour for various food applications.

Peanuts in Human Food Chain

The use of peanuts in the human food chain is very broad. Peanuts and peanut butter are used in candies, biscuits, cakes, ice cream, frozen confections, and ready-to-eat breakfast cereals. High-protein peanut flours are used commercially in bread, biscuits, cakes, muffins, and ground meat products, such as hamburgers, meat loaf, and sausages. Additionally, peanut proteins are used to replace milk proteins in cheese analogues, cheese spread, yogurt, and other fermented foods.

The American Dietetic Association (ADA) classifies peanuts and tree nuts as nutritious snacks, claiming that nuts are good sources of protein, carbohydrates, and essential minerals.[8] According to the Association's nutritional recommendations, the combination of a peanut butter sandwich and a glass of milk is considered a well-balanced meal, allegedly providing up to 40% of a child's daily nutrient requirements.

Table 1. Nuts of the World

Name	Source	Origin & History	Importance	Uses
Brazil Nut	The seed of the Brazil Nut tree	In Northern Brazil, the only region where it now grows	An important native food in the areas where it is grown. Also from the 30,000 and 40,000 metric tons are exported to the US and Europe	Snacks, ingredient in baking goods, confections, and nut mixures. The oil may be used in salads
Cashew Nut	The seed adhering to the cashew fruit	Introduced into India and Africa by the Portuguese	The fifth leading crop nut in the world, with an annual production of about 478,832 metric tons	Nut kernels are used as snacks, and as ingredients of baking goods and confections. Shell oil is used as a food and as a flavoring
Chestnut	The seed of the chestnut tree	Different species native to each of 4 areas: Europe, Africa, Asia, and the US	The sixth leading crop nut in the world, with an annual production of about 488,161 metric tons	Snacks; ingredients of confections, desserts, fritters, porridges, soups, stews, and stuffings

Table 1. Nuts of the World

Name	Source	Origin & History	Importance	Uses
Hazelnut	The seed of the hazel or filbert tree	Various species are native to Europe, Asia, and N. America	The seventh leading crop nut in the world, with an annual production of 561,000 metric tons	Snacks; ingredients of chocolates and other confections and desserts. Filbert oil is used in the manufacture of cosmetics and perfumes
Macadamia Nut	The seed of the macadamia tree	Brought to Hawaii, where it has prospered	One of the leading orchard crops of the Hawaiian islands, where about 18,210 short tons are produced annually	Snacks; ingredients of cakes, candy, and ice cream.
Pine Nut	The seeds of various species of pine trees	Trees are native to the areas noted under Species	The annual production in Northern Mexico and southwestern US averages 3,000 or more metric tons	Snacks; ingredients of baking goods, confections, desserts, and vegetarian dishes.
Pistachio Nut	The seed of the pistachio tree	Recently introduced to the central valley of California	The eighth leading crop nut in the world, with an annual production of about 220,490 metric tons	Snacks; ingredients of confections, desserts, ice cream

CHAPTER

2

Nut-Promoting Studies

The quest to reduce the epidemic of chronic disease among Americans has spurred many health and nutritional studies. These studies have attempted to show the impact of various diets and foodstuffs as either causes or remedies of certain diseases. Among the diseases studied, cardiovascular disease (CVD) has received the most attention because of its tremendous impact on the health of Americans.

According to federal epidemiological data, CVD is the nation's leading cause of death for both men and women among all racial and ethnic groups.[9] Approximately a million Americans die each year from CVD, accounting for 42% of all deaths. The financial toll of CVD is nearly $300 billion per year due to health and lost productivity costs from illness and death.

Cardiovascular diseases refers to diseases and conditions affecting the heart and blood vessels, principally high blood pressure, coronary heart disease (CHD), and stroke. CHD usually appears when cholesterol is deposited inside the walls of the heart's coronary arteries, which are the main suppliers of oxygen to the heart. When deposited there, it contributes to the formation of fatty blockages called plaque. This condition is known as arteriosclerosis or hardening of the arteries. Cholesterol can also be deposited within arteries elsewhere in the body, where it may contribute to the occurrence of stroke (from blocked arteries in the brain) and peripheral vascular disease (from arterial blockage in the legs).

LDL and HDL Debacle

In cardiovascular epidemiological and nutrition-based studies, researchers often use the terms "LDL" and "HDL". These terms are the primary factors used to measure the risk of heart disease, specifically CHD. They are also the factors used to measure the success of dietary regimens or specific nutrients in reducing the risks of CHD; thus understanding these terms helps us to properly evaluate the efficacy of nut-based health studies.

Figure 1. Atherosclerotic Plaque Formation

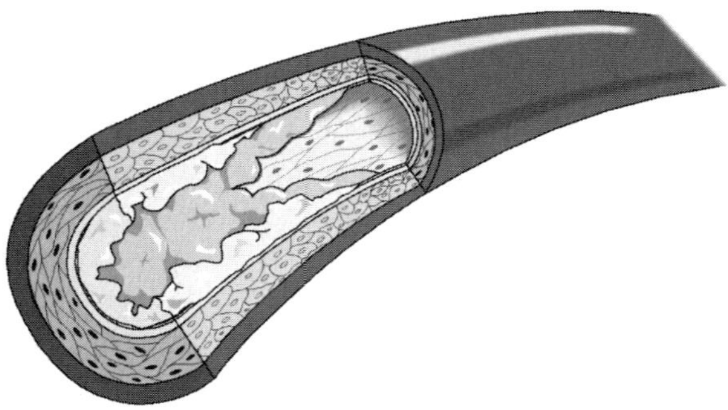

As noted, cholesterol is a major component in the etiology of CHD. However, in order to travel throughout the body, cholesterol and other lipid components must be wrapped inside water-soluble protein coats. These coats are called lipoproteins.

The primary cholesterol-carrying lipoproteins are low-density lipoproteins (LDL) and high-density lipoproteins (HDL). LDL is often referred to as the "bad" cholesterol because it appears to have a key role in depositing cholesterol within arteries, as it transports it and other fats from the liver to the body tissues. HDL is termed "good" cholesterol because it removes cholesterol from artery walls and carries it to the liver for excretion.

The biochemical distinction between LDL and HDL lies in the composition of each molecule. The more lipid contained in the lipoprotein molecule, the lower the density. The more protein contained in the lipoprotein, the higher the density. Both LDL and HDL transport lipids, but LDL is larger, lighter, and more lipid filled, while HDL is smaller and packaged with more protein. An elevated blood-LDL level is a risk factor for CHD, whereas elevated HDL concentrations are associated with low risk.

Nutritional Studies

Although other factors have been implicated as causes for CVD, the disease usually arises from poor lifestyle practices, such as smoking, excessive alcohol consumption, lack of exercise and diets that feature large daily intakes of fatty foods. Therefore, a consensus among health professionals is that behavior modification is a key to reducing the incidence of the disease.

Eliminating smoking and excessive alcohol are simple actions that have spurred little, if any, debate over the approaches used to resolve their health burden. If there are debates, they usually center on the controversial methods used to help people overcome addiction to these vices. For example, nicotine patches, pills, and chemical-laden chewing gums are methods used to help people break their smoking habits. However, some people believe that there are health dangers associated with these methods, and favor the use of a person's will power to overcome addiction.

Diet, on the other hand, has long been a controversial and confusing subject. There are hundreds of diets available, each staking a claim as the correct diet for humans. And, of course, exacerbating this dilemma is confusion among the medical and dietetic communities through the promotion of studies that allege that certain foodstuffs advance or prevent chronic diseases. This confusion stems from the differences of opinion among medical professionals.

For example, a common occurrence is that of two nutritionists or doctors, each boasting certifications from higher learning institutions, and yet disagreeing with each other about critical health and dietary issues. These disagreements are usually waged in the media through medical reports, health studies, and open health forums.

Such was the case in the so-called Great Nutrition Debate that was sponsored by the USDA in early-2000.[10] The authors of leading nutrition books, who were also medical practitioners, argued the issue of diet. Some authors advised the eating of meat, suggesting that meat is not unhealthy, while some opposed eating meat, claiming that meat is bad for your health. *So, which group is right? How do their disagreements impact the overall field of health, specifically nutrition?* This is the primary reason why key dietary issues must be resolved. Such issues include the identification of the proper foods, and the frequency of food intake.

There is, however, some agreement among health experts about the prevention of coronary heart disease. The common thread among most dietary recommendations is that people should reduce their intake of dietary fat, specifically saturated fat. Numerous health studies conducted throughout the 1970's and 1980's implicated saturated fat as the culprit for the increased incidence of heart disease.

Dietetic associations and food manufacturers responded to this research. Dietetic associations issued dietary recommendations, while the food industry responded by developing and marketing reduced-fat and fat-free foods. The thought was that such an effort would not only reduce the risk of heart disease, but would also curtail the rise in obesity. Obesity had risen to epidemic proportion over the past few decades. Large intakes of saturated fats were implicated as the cause for both heart disease and obesity.

Meanwhile, the federal government responded to this research by issuing dietary recommendations with respect to dietary fat. The Dietary Guidelines for Americans advised people to limit their intake of dietary fat to 30% of their daily food intake.[11] Surprisingly, neither the dietary recommendations nor the food industry's low fat products curtailed the rise in heart disease and obesity.

This led some medical scientists to shift their attention from dietary recommendations, in the general sense, to specific diets and nutrients. As a result, studies that measured the effectiveness of specific diets were conducted, as well as studies about the nutritional benefit of certain foodstuffs and food components.

Among the many diets studied, the Mediterranean Diet was and remains highly touted as a diet that is effective in reducing the risk of heart disease. As its name suggests, this diet is based upon the eating habits of people who live in the Mediterranean. According to studies, Mediterranean populations get more than 30% of their daily calories from fat; however, they rely on monounsaturated fat as their principal source of fat.

The Mediterranean Diet is deemed healthier than the high-fat American diet.[12] Healthy, in this sense, is defined as having lower rates of cancer, stroke and heart disease. Also, the life expectancy of people living in the Mediterranean is a few years longer than the average American.

Figure 2. Nut-Promoting Studies

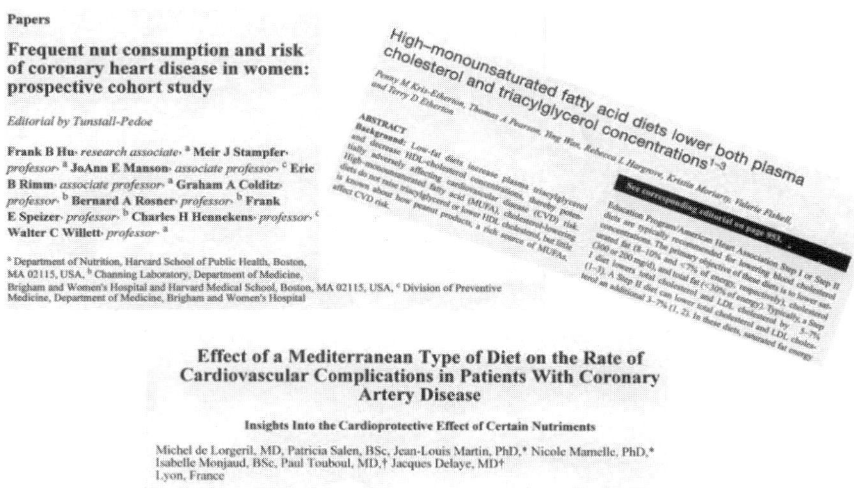

Papers

Frequent nut consumption and risk of coronary heart disease in women: prospective cohort study

Editorial by Tunstall-Pedoe

Frank B Hu, *research associate*, [a] Meir J Stampfer, *professor*, [a] JoAnn E Manson, *associate professor*, [c] Eric B Rimm, *associate professor*, [a] Graham A Colditz, *professor*, [b] Bernard A Rosner, *professor*, [b] Frank E Speizer, *professor*, [b] Charles H Hennekens, *professor*, [c] Walter C Willett, *professor* [a]

[a] Department of Nutrition, Harvard School of Public Health, Boston, MA 02115, USA, [b] Channing Laboratory, Department of Medicine, Brigham and Women's Hospital and Harvard Medical School, Boston, MA 02115, USA, [c] Division of Preventive Medicine, Department of Medicine, Brigham and Women's Hospital

High-monounsaturated fatty acid diets lower both plasma cholesterol and triacylglycerol concentrations[1-3]

Effect of a Mediterranean Type of Diet on the Rate of Cardiovascular Complications in Patients With Coronary Artery Disease

Insights Into the Cardioprotective Effect of Certain Nutriments

Michel de Lorgeril, MD, Patricia Salen, BSc, Jean-Louis Martin, PhD,* Nicole Mamelle, PhD,* Isabelle Monjaud, BSc, Paul Touboul, MD,† Jacques Delaye, MD†
Lyon, France

The Mediterranean diet features olive oil, nuts, seeds, and other grains. The significant intake of fat associated with this diet prompted medical scientists to consider the role that the type of fat has in heart disease, as opposed to the amount of fat. This consideration was also motivated by studies that suggested that the American "low fat" diet is rich in partially hydrogenated oils, and is therefore, high in unhealthy and harmful trans-fatty acids.

Trans-fatty acids are "hybrid-type" fatty acids that result when vegetable oils are infused with hydrogen atoms for the purpose of making the oils take on the characteristics of butter—having the look and storing capability of butter, but being something entirely different and dangerous.

Studies showed that the Mediterranean diet, or diets that are high in monounsaturated and polyunsaturated fats and low in saturated fats, reduced the risk of cardiovascular disease. For example, a study conducted at Penn State University tested the effects of two calorically-controlled diets on weight loss and cardiovascular disease.

One of the diets was low-fat, having less than 20% of the calories from fat; and one was higher in total fat, having 35% of calories from monounsaturated fat. Both groups lost an average of two pounds per week over the six-week study period, and preliminary results showed that both diets lowered total blood lipid and LDL-cholesterol levels.[13] This study, purportedly, served as evidence that a high-monounsaturated fat or "Mediterranean-style" diet is as good as a low-fat diet in lowering cardiovascular risk.

More focused studies into the health benefits of monounsaturated fat from certain foods, particularly nuts and peanuts, flooded the market. For example, several clinical studies that used a variety of nuts, including peanuts, walnuts and macadamia nuts, purportedly demonstrated that consumption of nuts lowered LDL cholesterol levels and possibly reduced the risks contributing to both fatal and non-fatal coronary heart disease.[14-17]

In one study, participants consumed one of five types of diets: a low-fat diet; one that included olive oil; one that included peanuts and peanut butter; one that included peanut oil; and a typical American diet. Participants who indulged the peanut diets were given the option of eating peanut butter bagel sandwiches, whole peanuts (as snacks), or peanut oil (in their salad).

The results purportedly showed that the diets that included peanuts and peanut butter; peanut oil; and olive oil lowered total cholesterol and LDL-cholesterol levels. Furthermore, each of these three diets lowered triglyceride levels, but did not lower the HDL cholesterol. The low-fat diet was successful in lowering LDL cholesterol levels, but it also lowered "good" HDL cholesterol and increased triglyceride levels.[18]

In yet another study, 500 calories of peanuts were either added to the regular diets of participants; substituted in the diet for other fat; or eaten freely. The results were the same in that both men and women favored the high satiety of peanuts. According to the study, those who added peanuts to their regular diet, or substituted peanuts for other fats, had lowered their triglyceride levels.[19]

According to researchers, snacks of peanuts and peanut butter produced more eating satisfaction and feelings of fullness than high-carbohydrate snacks, such as rice cakes. Furthermore, the study purported that subjects who were fed the peanut snacks self-adjusted their caloric intakes, so they did not add extra calories to their daily diets.[20]

Another study purportedly found a linear relationship between the risk of CHD and nut consumption. The study suggested that people who ate nuts more than 5 times a week decreased their risk of heart disease by over 50 percent, and those who ate nuts 1 to 4 times per week decreased their risk by 27 percent.[21]

A so-called landmark study of approximately 27,000 Seventh-Day Adventists in California examined the relationship between 65 different foods and coronary heart disease. Researchers concluded that among the foods studied, nuts had the strongest protective effect against the risk of fatal heart disease.[22]

A study at Penn State University purportedly found that peanut eaters consistently tended to have higher levels of key nutrients and overall healthier diets than their non-peanut eating counterparts. Additionally, the body mass index (a weight measurement criteria) of peanut eaters was found to be favorable to that of non-peanut eaters.[23]

Researchers from the Harvard School of Public Health suggested that eating just two servings of peanuts and nuts per week may decrease the risk of having another coronary event (heart attack) among people who had survived a heart attack. Researchers followed participants in the CARE trial over 4 years and purportedly found that compared to those who rarely or never consumed nuts, subjects who consumed two or more servings of peanuts and nuts per week decreased their risk of heart disease by 25%.[24]

A study published in the March 2000 issue of the Journal of the American Dietetic Association, purported that incorporating approximately 3/4 cups of pecans into a regular diet on a daily basis might significantly reduce LDL-cholesterol levels.[25] This finding was the result of an eight-week study by New Mexico State University. It was the first nutritional study dedicated to pecans.

In this study, nineteen participants with normal cholesterol levels were selected from the New Mexico area. Nine were randomly assigned to the control group, who followed their typical diet and ate no pecans or other tree nuts for the duration of the study. The other ten participants were randomly assigned to the pecan group and instructed to eat 68 grams (3/4 cup) of pecans a day—either out of hand or added to their favorite recipes.

After four weeks, the pecan group had lowered their LDL-cholesterol by 10 percent, as well as their total cholesterol despite an increased intake of monounsaturated fat, polyunsaturated fat and insoluble fiber. The pecan study was supported by funding from the New Mexico State University Agricultural Experiment Station in Las Cruces, N.M., and by a grant from the Western Pecan Growers Association.

Women have also been the subjects of studies featuring nut consumption. In one study, researchers at the Harvard School of Public Health purported that frequent consumption of peanuts and nuts was associated with a lowered risk of coronary heart disease.[26] In this study, the Nurses Health Study, the eating habits and health outcomes of over 86,000 women, ages 34-59, were followed for almost 20 years. After adjusting for age, smoking, and other known risk factors for CHD, the purported result was that women who ate more than five servings of nuts and peanuts per week decreased their risk of heart disease by approximately one third, compared to women who rarely or never ate nuts.

Another study, the Iowa Women's Study, included approximately 34,000 post-menopausal women with no cardiovascular disease. The study purportedly found that higher levels of nut consumption were related to lower risks of death from heart disease.[27]

The diets and occurrence of cardiac death of approximately 22,000 male physicians were studied, and preliminary results suggested that as nut consumption increased, the risk of cardiac death decreased.[28] According to the study, this inverse relationship between cardiac death and consumption of nuts and peanuts persisted after controlling for age, exercise, hypertension, cholesterol, smoking, diabetes, use of alcohol, and other dietary habits.

Some researchers have gone as far as to suggest that nuts contain anticarcinogen properties, specifically the phytosterol, beta-sitosterol (SIT). According to written speculations, SIT might inhibit cancer growth.[29] Researchers at New York State University in Buffalo examined the SIT content of peanuts, peanut butter, peanut flour and peanut oil and found that the SIT content varied from 44 mg SIT/100 gm (peanut flour) to 191 mg SIT/100 gm (unrefined peanut oil). Snack peanuts contain 160 mg SIT/100 gm and peanut butter contains approximately 120 mg SIT/100 gm.

As is customary with suggestive findings, more research is required to confirm the anticarcinogenic properties in peanuts, but these published speculations, most likely, have been enough to send people racing to gobble down bags of peanuts. There should be an ethical stipulation that studies not be released to the media until their findings are scientifically confirmed.

Studies such as those presented in this chapter appear to confirm that nuts are healthy foods to eat. Such an appearance is fortified by the reputations of the education and scientific institutions that conducted them. This, combined with the powerful media, has influenced people to consume nuts.

Despite the success of nut-promoting studies in the media, the studies, themselves, are grossly insufficient in proving that nuts are healthy foods for humans. In the next chapter, the validity and relevancy of these studies are challenged. And, the core factors that contribute to heart disease are addressed.

CHAPTER

3

Studies' Questioned

From the outset, we must note that health-related studies register economic and social impacts. Economically, studies that seek to measure the effectiveness of certain foods and drugs usually result in financial gain for the companies that develop, harvest, and market those products. For example, if you knew that a certain food or drug might decrease the signs of aging, would you hesitate to purchase the product? Most people would dart to the market to get that product. Of course, many have done exactly that with products that boast miraculous benefits.

The social implication caused by health-related studies is that people are either benefactors of the advice generated from the studies or they are not. When they do not benefit, they are usually robbed of money and, in some cases, life. When losses are experienced, it compromises the public's confidence in the scientific community. As it now stands, a growing number of people believe that science has become a tool for commerce rather than a legitimate means through which the quality of life is continuously improved.

Will nut-promoting studies produce health benefits for the population or will they cause people to advance further down the road of disease and early mortality? This question is addressed in this chapter, as the validity of these studies is examined.

The researchers' purpose for conducting the nut-promoting studies was to show that nuts are healthy foods, and therefore, should be eaten. There are several dangerous flaws in the evidence that purportedly justifies nut consumption. These flaws are manifested in the general approach to health, and in the lack of pertinent information about the causes of heart disease.

Miracle Approach to Health

The foremost flaw of the nut-promoting studies is in the overall approach to disease prevention upon which the studies were based. Health researchers often engage studies from the premise that a single nutrient is responsible for disease, combined with the notion that there exist a miracle food that can prevent disease. This is reminiscent of the deadly debacle that lead to the formation of the Food and Drug Administration. Nostrum makers and other unscrupulous, money-driven persons had marketed adulterated foods, nostrums, and other harmful substances, which they declared delivered miraculous health benefits.[30] Quackery is the name given to this practice.

During that period, people were under the scourge of deadly infectious, and degenerative diseases, so products that boasted miraculous claims attracted large followings. Many people were injured after following such advice, particularly after consuming the "miracle" substances.

The FDA first intervened by prohibiting interstate commerce of misbranded and adulterated foods, drinks and drugs.[31] Years later, the agency established a criteria to prevent misleading claims by food and drug manufacturers.[32] To date, health-related claims are required to be scientifically proven before they are FDA-approved and sent to the marketplace.

However, after examining the current health climate, it is evident that the practice of rendering misleading claims has never been aborted, in spite of the FDA's intervention. The incidence of chronic disease has remained high and companies continue to market miracle foods, nostrums, drugs, and other substances. In fact, the FDA has been the principal exponent for this "miracle" substance approach. So-called medical professionals, nutritionists, and quacks, alike, are standing on the unproven and volatile premise that a miracle food, drug, potion or lotion exist. The only difference between the pre-FDA era and today is that their positions are supported by so-called scientific health studies.

These institutions that engage bogus research have joined forces with bio-pharmaceutical companies to concoct drugs that are touted as solutions to numerous diet-related diseases.[33] Despite these efforts, disease is still rampant and the very drugs, themselves, have exacerbated the onslaught of illness. We are accustomed to seeing FDA-approved drugs pulled off the market after causing significant injury and death to consumers.[34] This frequent occurrence makes the scientific studies, which purportedly established the validity of the drugs, suspect. Some people have even called such studies advertisements.[35]

Meanwhile, nutritional companies continue to concoct so-called health foods that have caused similar harm. And, throughout this debacle, nutritionists continue to herald individual foods or food components as "miracle" substances.

The growing number of research-based nutrition institutions and would-be nutritionists has corrupted the market with so-called studies. Most of these studies are confusing, based upon faulty research and profit driven. For example, earlier research purported that fiber reduces the risks of colon cancer. When this news hit the media, fiber-based foods, supplements and other concoctions flooded the market. Studies later released, countered this research, and suggested that fiber had nothing to do with reducing colon cancer risks.

These contradictory studies triggered a war—a war that was played out in the public—between proponents and opponents of fiber. Organizations representing nurses, dieticians, and other health practitioners were involved in this literary fist-a-cuffs. There were no winners, but consumers were the losers.

The fiber debacle, unfortunately, is one of many dietary myths and counter-myths that the public has had to contend with. Health claims for oats, orange juice, and margarine have been opposed by other research. In the research arena, what's good today might be bad tomorrow, and what was good yesterday is no longer good today. In the public arena, responding to this advice is difficult. Consumers lose money, health, and confidence.

Scientific health studies that tout products are, undoubtedly, advertisements because the revenues of companies that market these *miracle* products are substantially increased. In many cases, food companies fund such studies through grant programs, which they offer to higher education and health institutions. An example of this, as mentioned in the previous chapter, was the funding of New Mexico State University's pecan study by the Western Pecan Growers Association. *How can fair and unbiased results be expected?* This deceitful conduct was disguised as bona-fide research and the "favorable" results circulated through the media, spurring the purchase of pecans.

The danger with this "miracle substance" approach is that it is not relevant to securing good health. Good health does not hinge on nutrients, alone. Consumption of required nutrients is essential; however, it only represents one of several areas or pillars that comprise a healthy diet. Another pillar is the frequency of food intake. In fact, the greater evidence as to the root cause of disease lies in this area. This fact leads us to another flaw contained in the nut-promoting health studies—the omission of obesity as a leading risk factor for CHD.

What about Obesity?

As previously stated, overeating is a major factor driving the chronic disease epidemic. This is demonstrated by the astronomical rise in obesity, which is also epidemic. Obesity is a risk factor for nearly every chronic disease, especially heart disease. The rise in obesity corresponds to the rise in heart disease risks and heart failure. This fact confirms that the association of obesity and heart disease is greater than the alleged connection between dietary fat and heart disease. *How is this so?*

Obesity occurs from the accumulation of fat in the body. This fat, however, does not only come from the consumption of dietary fat. All nutrients, including protein and starch, consumed in excess of the body's needs are converted to fat and stored in body tissue. This fat later metabolizes and enters the blood stream, increasing the risks of heart disease.

Nothing More Than Crash Diets

The short duration of the nut-promoting studies represents a major flaw that renders such studies null and void. These studies were not engaged long enough to justify a finding. Most studies were only conducted over several weeks, except those in which the findings were extrapolated from periodic health surveys (i.e. Nurses Health Study).

Short-term studies are inadequate in proving the health benefit of nuts or any food or drug. *Why*? Any drastic change in a person's diet registers immediate observable changes, whether the person is overweight or healthy. In this respect, the studies are no more than crash diets.

What are crash diets? They are diets that feature particular foods or food components, with the goal of bringing about immediate results, such as weight loss. For this reason, crash diets are, generally, nutritionally imbalanced. They also do not achieve long-term results—whether the intended result is weight loss or a reduced blood-lipid level.

Why would health institutions choose to conduct studies over such a short duration? Is it that they know that after a certain time, the body begins to respond to that diet, and that such a response determines the true effectiveness of that diet? In most cases, after 6 to 8 weeks, the body adapts and most people find the weight and other discouraging ailments returning. This is more likely to happen when the diet does not contain consumption parameters, such as eating once a day. Over consumption of any type of food will produce weight gain.

Furthermore, the nut-promoting studies contained little, if any, follow-up, which prevents us from knowing how the participants fared months or years later. *Did their blood-lipid and LDL levels eventually rise again? Did nuts really benefit them?* Proper follow-up is very important. Unfortunately, it has been omitted from most studies.

We must consider the fact that obesity and heart disease are not conditions that are instantly acquired. They are metabolic disorders that result from a lengthy duration of poor lifestyle and dietary habits. So, health studies must also be long-term to show the true impact of a new dietary regimen. For a researcher to suggest that nuts can miraculously eliminate chronic health conditions in a few weeks is deceptive. The remedy for chronic diseases such as heart disease must include a comprehensive approach—diet and behavior modifications.

Aim of Food

A flaw that dismantles the very foundation of the nut-promoting studies is the omission of the overall aim of food. The aim of food is not disease prevention in as much as it is the prolongation of life. Therefore, studies that use specific foods to address specific diseases are flawed from the outset.

For example, findings in the Nurses Health Study suggested that nurses who ate nuts five times a week did not die from heart disease as early as those who did not consume nuts.[26] A reduction in the risk of heart disease is alleged, but longevity is subtly implied. Yet, increased longevity was not the goal of the study. *Does "reduced risk" mean that the nurses who ate nuts will not eventually die from heart disease or any other disease—within the next year or two?* No, it doesn't. *Does it mean that they will exceed life expectancy?* No, it doesn't. *So, what does reduced-risk actually connote in this study?*

Hidden Variables

The Nurses Health Study documented several interesting points, which raises questions about its conclusions. One point was that the consumption of vegetables and fruits in both groups—those who ate nuts frequently and those who ate no nuts—were similar. The consumption of vegetables and fruits have long been established as foods that reduce the incidence of chronic disease, especially heart disease.

Another point was that the women who consumed nuts ate less meat than the women who rarely ate nuts. Again, meat consumption is considered a risk factor for heart disease and other chronic diseases. *So, was it the reduction of meat consumption that reduced the risk of heart disease or was it frequent nut consumption? Was it the consumption of meat that increased the risk of heart disease for women who ate fewer nuts, or was it that they ate fewer nuts that increased their risk for heart disease?*

These variables make the findings of the Nurses Health Study very suspect. When they are considered, it is quite evident that this study did not prove that nuts reduced the risk of heart disease.

Other Pathways to Heart Disease

Another omission intrinsic in the nut-promoting studies is the fact that there are several pathways to heart disease. In the case of most of the studies, the often-touted result was decreased LDL levels; but other conditions create high LDL levels and serve as risk factors for heart disease.

For example, thyroid disease, diabetes, osteoporosis, stress, and menopause are also risk factors for heart disease. Few nut-promoting studies assessed the participants for any of these conditions. What is the impact of nut consumption on these health conditions? How does consuming nuts really intervene in heart disease? Biological underpinnings prove they don't intervene. *A better question, however, is how does nut consumption contribute to any of the other diseases?*

Nut Poison's Contribution to Disease

A host of diseases stem from the consumption of plant toxins, several of which are contained in nuts. This subject is taken up in the next chapter, but suffice to state that this fact unveils the most dangerous flaw of nut-promoting studies—the absence of biochemical research that shows that nuts contain toxins that are harmful to humans when ingested.[36] Such data is plentiful and the fact that it was not considered in any of the studies is indicative of the abuse of science by profit-seeking industries.

May and May Not

A less noticeable flaw in nearly all studies is the use of terms that demonstrated the unwillingness of researchers to commit to their findings. Actually, the studies made no claims, but merely implied or suggested definite outcomes, findings, and conclusions. Nothing was actually affirmed in any study. For example, all studies used the term "may" or "might" (i.e. "may reduce risk").

The use of such terms show that despite the researchers' purported findings, none were willing to emphatically state that nuts reduced the risk of heart disease. They preferred to use speculative terminology. Perhaps they wanted to avoid repercussions from people who did not experience the purported benefits after following the advice to consume nuts.

Who knows why speculations are disguised as definite outcomes? As it stands, evasive and suggestive language is skillfully inserted into scientific studies. Researchers are able to get away with using obscured lingo because the reputation of their institutions subtly validates their studies. Who would dare think that research coming from Harvard University is unfounded, speculative, and outright bogus? Few people would think such, although this is evident in nut-promoting studies.

Verdict: Not Relevant

Research that only focuses on the lipid content of certain foods is inadequate in proving a food beneficial to humans. It can safely be concluded that nut-promoting studies deceive people because the studies purport health advantages that are nothing more than speculations, yet imply that they are factual. Additionally, the studies omit the disadvantages or dangers associated with ingesting nut poisons. As such, these studies follow the pre-FDA tradition, wherein notoriously false claims are made for profit's sake.

In the case of nuts, it's ironic that the greater disadvantage or harm caused by nut consumption is the very thing that the studies suggest nuts prevent—heart disease. Nuts are not the villains, but ignorance about the biochemical nature of foodstuffs, and the animals that are better equipped to consume them, are among the principle causes of diet-related diseases. The next two chapters cover these areas, and prove that the Honorable Elijah Muhammad is correct when stating that nuts are unfit for human consumption.

CHAPTER

4

Digestive Differences

The main purpose of the digestive system is to break down food into the components necessary for use by the biological cell—the basic unit of life. Cells reproduce to form tissue; tissue construct organs; and, organs make up the body. Through it all, it is the biological cell that needs the material and energy to handle its vital processes. This material and energy is provided through food.

Food is degraded by mechanical and chemical processes. Mechanical processes include chewing and churning—the peristaltic actions of muscular organs, such as the esophagus, stomach and intestines. Chemical processes are the actions of the digestive juices on food. Digestive juices sever the bonds of the molecules that compose the food, reducing the molecules to their basic elements.

The coordinated actions of several body organs are responsible for digestion, and are systematically termed, the digestive system. Illustratively, the digestive process mirrors a "disassembly line", wherein the digestive organs and digestive juices combine to disassemble the ingested food.

The major nutrients of food that require digestion are proteins, starches, and fats. These large molecules are broken down into smaller units or their basic building blocks. Proteins are degraded to amino acids; starch, a polysaccharide, is broken down into monosaccharides or simple sugars; and fats are dismantled into smaller units, as well. These nutrients are then absorbed into the bloodstream, and made available to the cells.

Most food—for all living creatures—is comprised of protein, lipids, and carbohydrates, yet there are distinct differences among the creatures that rely on this food to sustain their lives. The distinct physiological differences among mammals, such as those between humans and birds, are indicative of the anatomical differences and processes that support the life of each group. The most studied of these differences is digestion. This is because digestion is essential to health; and therefore, to life. The life of any creature is dependent upon that creature's ability to obtain and efficiently use food.

Does the physiological difference among digestive systems mean that there are biochemical differences among foodstuffs that support the life of each creature? It certainly does. Foodstuffs are different in biochemical structure, and their degradation, which also includes the elimination of poisons, comes through several pathways. As already noted, one pathway is the action of digestive organs and juices. The other is the use of external processing methods, such as cooking.

We are aware that animals, generally, eat their food raw. Humans prefer cooked food. Cooking changes a food's biochemical structure by denaturing its molecules. It also rids the food of numerous poisons, which are not foreign components, but complex proteins, carbohydrates, and lipids.

Of course, all foods require digestion; however, there are some foods that also require external processing before they can be effectively digested. In fact, except for fruit, most of the natural foods eaten by humans require external processing. For example, vegetables contain concentrated nutrients that can only be unleashed through cooking. When vegetables are eaten in their raw stages, the nutrients are not totally accessible to us.

There are also natural foods that neither external processing nor normal digestive action can render suitable for use by the human body. The food, however, is not the blame. In such cases, the human digestive system is not adapted or designed to digest these foods. Simply stated, the human digestive system lacks the organs, digestive juices and functionality necessary to digest such foods.

Consequently, when these foods are eaten, they render an anti-nutritional effect. This adverse effect causes stress to the digestive system as it attempts to manage the complex components that comprise the food. Additionally, numerous molecular disruptions occur. Sickness, disease, and death are the ultimate consequences of ingesting such foods.

Not only are proteins, lipids, and carbohydrates the major nutrients in food, they are also the major antinutrients. The terms—proteins, lipids, and carbohydrates—represent three broad categories of molecules. Each category contains sub-molecules. These sub-molecules have the same core structure, but different peripheral structures and binding properties.

It is the core structure that designates them to that category; however, the peripheral structures and binding properties make each sub-molecule unique. This uniqueness determines the molecules' digestibility. Many people are unaware of this.

For example, some people think that there is only one specific protein, and as such, assume that the protein in foods is the same—only differing in amount. This is not so. There are many types of proteins. *How is this?*

Proteins are similar only in that they are comprised of amino acids; however, the arrangement of the amino acids, combined with the type of bonds that connect them, determine the quality of the protein, as well as whether or not it can be denatured and digested.

Some proteins are complex or rich because they have strong bonds. Simple proteins contain bonds that are easily denatured by human digestive enzymes. Therefore, some proteins are degradable by digestive enzymes and some are not. Those that are not degradable usually render antinutritional effects by serving as poison. Such poisons are often classified as *naturally-occurring* toxins.

The Honorable Elijah Muhammad uses the word "poison" when referring to these components, because this is most accurate in describing their adverse health impact. Also, the use of other terms, specifically "anti-nutrient", subversively blames the food for the adverse reaction. This permits poisonous foods to remain in the food chain, while food manufacturers employ various processing methods to rid the food of its "villain" substances—allegedly making the food suitable for our consumption. This practice has been engaged for centuries, and has allowed extremely complex foods, particularly animal food, to be fed to humans.

Contrarily, the term "poison" denotes danger. Something that is dangerous must either be handled with caution or not at all. If the foods that are heavily laden with these harmful substances were labeled poisonous, many of them would not be on the market. As it stands, poisonous foods persist throughout the human food chain.

A noteworthy point is that food manufacturers usually use toxic chemicals to degrade impermeable food components. In most cases, the food's natural poisons are fortified with chemical poisons, making the food more dangerous. This approach is characteristic of an attempt to place a round peg into a square hole. Food manufacturers force animal food into the human food chain, and then influence, via advertisements, people to eat foods that are dangerous to their health. This practice is among the many reasons why a distinction among foods is necessary.

The Honorable Elijah Muhammad brings this vitally important distinction to the forefront of human nutrition, and declares it essential to producing healthier and longer human life spans. In opposition to popular nutritional recommendations, He states that nuts are not fit for human consumption, but for birds, which possess the digestive systems suited to digest nuts. His position warrants consideration; so the following sections compare the bird and the human digestive systems.

Bird Digestive System

Birds have obvious features that distinguish them from humans. They are lower creatures, quite physically smaller, usually chirp, and are known to fly. There are also obvious digestive differences—birds lack teeth and have beaks. Just as important, is the fact that birds do not cook their food, as they prefer raw seeds, grains, nuts, and insects. These things, alone, are sufficient to raise the argument against the consumption of nuts by humans.

Physiologically, the digestive process of birds is designed for maximum utilization of food in a short timeframe.[37] Prolonged food digestion, such as that which occurs in humans, would temporarily incapacitate birds, making them vulnerable to predators. Birds can digest a meal within several hours. Some frugivorous birds digest seeds and nuts in 20 to 30 minutes. On the other hand, it is generally known that humans have difficulty digesting nuts. Nuts are usually found intact in human stool, confirming that they are not digestible.

Birds possess digestive organs that enable them to digest dense and complex nutrients such as nuts and seeds. These organs are additions to a digestive tract that is, functionally, similar to humans. The extra digestive organs that birds possess include a *crop*, an *extra stomach* (equaling two stomachs), and a *cloaca*. The other digestive organs that mirror those of humans, include a small intestine, colon, and stomach, as well as the accessory digestive organs—pancreas, kidneys, etc.

Digestion in the bird begins after food is seized by its beak, and makes its way through the beak cavity. The beak is the vital organ birds use to obtain food. Without it, birds cannot survive. The food is coarsely ground by the beak's sharp edges, and is then moved by the tongue to the pharynx, where it is swallowed.

Figure 3. Various Birds

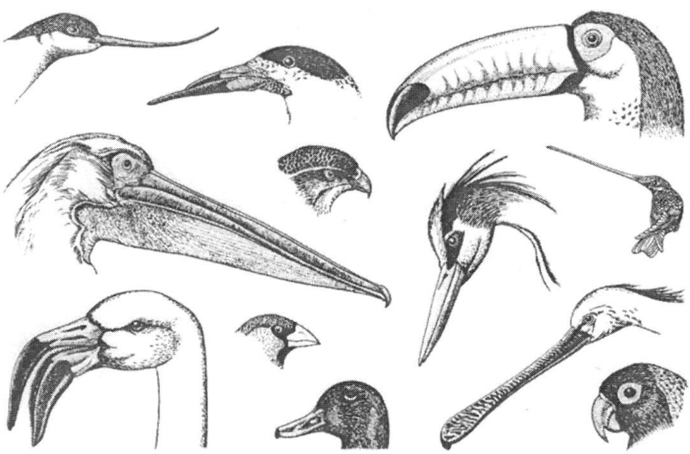

The bird's swallowing function is not a peristaltic act because of the absence of a soft palate and constrictor muscle in the pharynx. Birds use their hard plated tongues to press the food into the mouth-like opening of the esophagus. Additionally, there is a passive swallowing. Birds, through lifting their heads and reducing pressure in the esophagus, allow gravity to move food and water to the stomach.

In the esophagus, the food is managed by peristaltic contractions and guided toward the crop. The crop is represented by an out-pouching of the esophagus wall. Only after filling the stomach is the swallowed food deposited in the crop. So, the crop's principle function is to store food. When room is available in the stomach, the crop is gradually emptied through peristaltic action, refilling the stomach.

The crop is also used when birds are obtaining food for their young. In this manner, the crop is used to store food for transport. The food is then regurgitated to feed the nestlings.

While in the crop, there is a softening and swelling of the grain food by means of the beak saliva that accompanied it as it made its way into the crop, and also by means of the secretions of the esophagus and crop glands. Swelling and softening, but no digestion, takes place in the crop. After passing the esophagus and the crop, the swollen and softened food reaches the stomach.

The stomach of birds is multichambered, consisting of two parts: the glandular stomach and the muscular stomach. They are arranged one behind the other. The glandular stomach, known as the proventriculus, is considered the real stomach because it mirrors the stomach found in monogastric animals, wherein gastric juices are secreted to act upon the food. It is in this stomach where the food is made suitable for the next stage of the digestion process.

We must, however, note that the bird's glandular stomach digestive acids are more powerful than the gastric acid contained in the human stomach. The bird's stomach secretes a pepsin-hydrochloric acid that is capable of dissolving complex materials, such as bones and fish fins.

After the food leaves the glandular stomach, it enters the muscular stomach. The muscular stomach, known as the ventriculus is colloquially called the *"gizzard"*. It is considered the bird's pulverizing apparatus, serving as a chewing stomach that grinds the nuts and other hard foodstuffs.

The gizzard is characterized by its unique construction and digestive function. Anatomically, the gizzard is a highly muscular organ that is lined with a tough, abrasive keratin-like material. Keratin is a structural protein that the body produces to construct durable body parts such as nails and hair. Anyone who has eaten a gizzard knows that it is very tough to chew, and is never fully masticated. This is proof of the gizzard's extraordinary toughness.

The gizzard's tough construction is necessary because in order for birds to degrade hard foodstuffs, such as nuts, they must first ingest acid resistant pebbles, granite stones, or sand stones—all commonly referred to as *grit*. The word *grit* is synonymous with sand, as its action is similar to that of sandpaper, which is used to grind away tough materials. The gizzard's keratin-like lining can withstand the grinding of sand, stones, glass, and other sharp materials ingested by birds. It allows birds to process relatively large volumes of food each day.

It is also important to note that there has been a debate among aviculturists with respect to the type of grit used in the birds' (specifically, chickens') diets. Some use shell grit and cuttlefish bone, because they supply calcium, while aiding the digestive process. However, others refrain from the use of these materials because they are not sufficient for the task of grinding up hard grains. Seed kernels, such as nuts, are hard and require harder grit to degrade. They have also found that when left alone, birds naturally consume the appropriate materials needed to aid in the degradation of dense foods such as nuts, seeds and grains. They will usually choose small stones and other hard materials.

Functionally, the propulsion activity of the gizzard is an intrinsic part of the bird's ability to degrade seeds and nuts. The contraction force of the gizzard is extremely powerful. For example, a turkey's gizzard is so powerful that it is capable of crushing walnuts and glass balls. It can also effectively manage metal particles. The high pressure, combined with the action of grit upon the foodstuffs, pulverizes the food, making it suitable for the digestive enzymes in the intestines to effectively dismantle the chemical bonds.

This aspect is very important because foods such as nuts contain heat stable proteins that cannot be degraded by heat treatment or human digestive juices. This subject will be covered in the next chapter, but consider this question: *When humans eat nuts—the same nuts as birds—how can we expect to gain nutrition from nuts without having the same digestive organs required for the bird to gain nutrition from those very nuts?*

Figure 4. Avian Digestive System

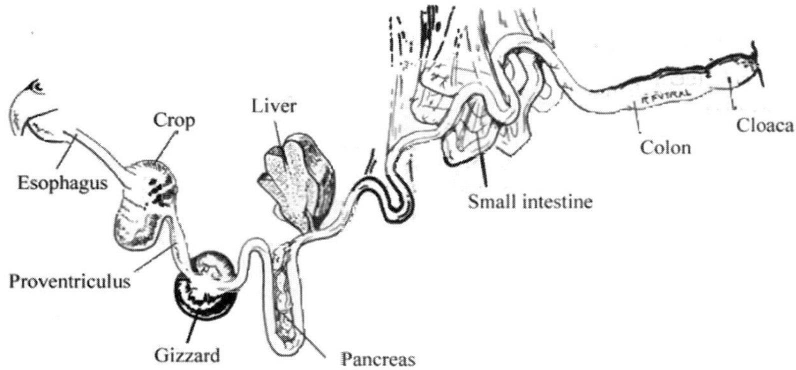

Continuing, the finely macerated food passes by peristalsis out of the gizzard into the intestines. Although the activities of the bird's intestines are similar to that of humans, the bird's intestinal length is much shorter in relation to the human's. The bird, however, compensates for the short intestinal length through the gizzard's pulverizing activity. The extremely denatured food that passes from the gizzard allows for expedient digestion and absorption in the small intestines.

The small intestine is where digestion and absorption of food occur. The liver and pancreas connect to the duodenum and secrete bile and pancreatic juices into the small intestines. These juices emulsify fats, and digest carbohydrates, proteins and fats. Nutrients are absorbed through the intestinal wall and pass into the kidneys. After processing in the kidneys, the nutrients are distributed throughout the body.

The indigestible remains pass from the small intestines into either the colon or the cloaca. Some birds have both organs, as previously noted. The cloaca is a compartment positioned aside the colon that houses large quantities of bacteria, which assist in the break down of complex carbohydrates. Water is also absorbed in the cloaca.

Whether the food enters the cloaca or the colon depends on the composition of the feces. If the feces contain significant quantities of cellulose and other fibers, it must pass through the cloaca. After the material is handled in the cloaca, it passes through the colon for elimination. Feces that do not contain complex carbohydrates and other fibers pass directly to the colon.

We must also note that the bird's colon is, functionally, different from the human colon. The bird's colon corresponds, physiologically, to the human rectum. The breakdown of complex carbohydrates that takes place in the human colon is performed in the bird's cloaca.

Human Digestive System

The human digestive system consists of a hollow tube that begins at the mouth and extends to the anus. Organs of the digestive tract include the mouth, pharynx, esophagus, stomach, small intestine, colon, and anus. The organs that aid the digestive process consist of the salivary glands, gall bladder, liver, and pancreas. They assist in the digestive process by secreting substances, such as enzymes and acid juices, which degrade food.

Our tongues and teeth, as well as a specific digestive enzyme, salivary amylase, begin the digestive process. Salivary amylase is an enzyme that starts the chemical digestion of starch, which among other purposes, permits us to enjoy the taste of food on our palates.

After the food is thoroughly chewed (mixed with saliva), it is pushed into the pharynx, and passes through the esophagus—the act of swallowing. Peristaltic contractions move the food through the esophagus into the stomach.

While in the stomach, the food bolus under goes a great deal of churning and mixing movements. The food bolus is also acted upon by an array of chemicals that turns it into a substance called, "chyme". Gastrin (a hormone), mucus, hydrochloric acid, and several protein-digesting enzymes (pepsinogen and renin) are secreted into the stomach to further degrade the food. These substances prepare the chyme for absorption in the small intestines.

Gastrin and hydrochloric acid are released into the stomach to help produce the environment that enables pepsin and renin to digest proteins. Besides protein digestion, very little digestion occurs in the stomach. Once chyme is produced, peristalsis begins in the lower half of the stomach and forces the chyme through an opening (pyloric sphincter) that leads to the small intestine.

Figure 5. Human Digestive System

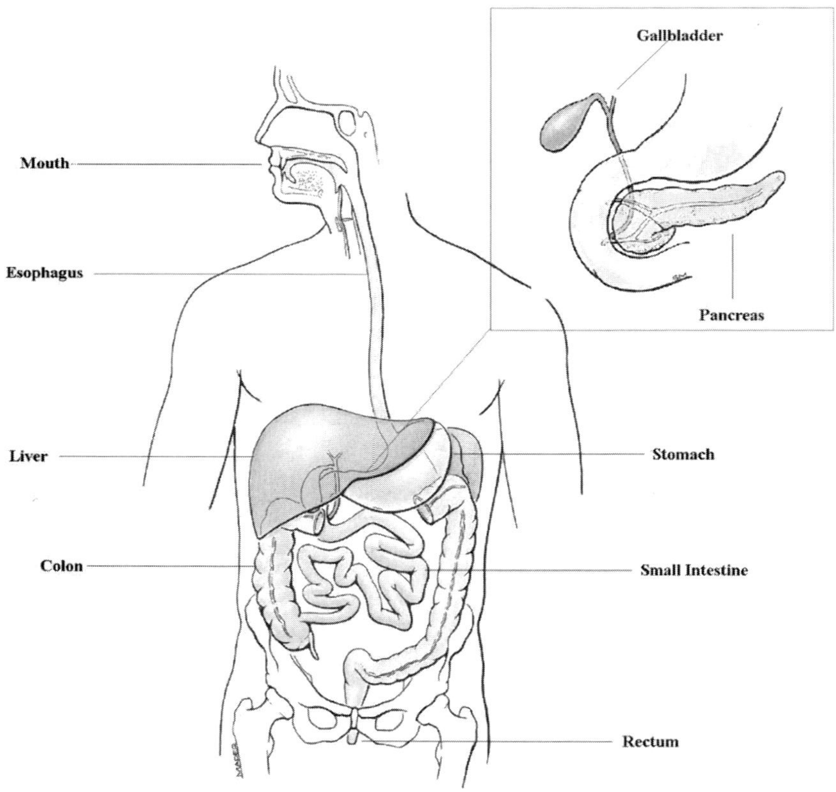

The passage of chyme into the small intestine is regulated to avoid an overflow of the duodenum; thus, only small amounts can enter at a time. It takes several hours for the stomach to completely empty chyme into the small intestine. The pancreas secretes pancreatic fluid that breaks down proteins, fats, and starches. Intestinal juice secreted by the small intestine also contains enzymes that complete the process begun by the pancreatic fluid. Bile is secreted by the liver to aid the digestion of fats.

The degraded nutrients are transported through the wall of the small intestine and taken into the body. Nutrients—amino acids, carbohydrates, and minerals—are transferred to the liver. Most fats are picked up by the lymphatic system. The undigested material enters the colon where it forms a solid mass or feces. Water, salts, and vitamins are absorbed in the colon. The feces are pushed to the rectum and passes through the anus.

The human digestion process is a monumental event, requiring 24 or more hours for a meal to completely digest. Depending upon the quality of the food, it takes the stomach approximately 4 hours to pass the food to the small intestines. Approximately 8 hours are required for the small intestine to digest and absorb the nutrients. The large intestine requires approximately 12 hours to complete its functions.

A Priority Consideration

In this comparison—between the human and bird digestive systems—several differences have been noted, which must be considered when determining the foods that are fit for either creature. The major differences are the organs and the digestive processes required by each creature to digest certain foodstuffs. Additionally, the overall digestive timeframe is very notable. For example, birds have the organs that allow them to process nuts and seeds in a matter of hours. On the other hand, humans require 24 hours to digest foods that are digestible, not to think of indigestible foods, such as nuts.

Unlike humans, birds are not eager to eat human food or sit at our dinner tables. Furthermore, if presented with a bowl of sunflower seeds and a bowl of chicken noodle soup, birds would opt for the seeds. The soup is not suitable to meet the nutritional demands of birds. And, although nuts are being touted as nutritious human food, they are not suited to meet the nutritional demands of humans. Nuts are too complex for the human digestive system. The harm that results from ingesting nuts outweighs any purported nutritional benefit.

CHAPTER

5

Nut Poisons Described

The digestive systems of all life forms determine and define the type of materials that are eligible for digestion by them. The comparison of the human and avian digestive systems presented in the previous chapter is evidence of this. Many more examples could easily be shown, as there are thousands of creatures that gain nutrition through unique digestive systems and eating patterns.

Most of us can agree that the human digestive tract is quite different from that of birds, cattle and insects. It is also obvious that the eating patterns of these creatures are different from the eating patterns of humans. Unfortunately, we can also agree that humans eat some of the same foods consumed by birds, cattle, and insects despite these anatomical differences.

This confirms that there is a gross lack of understanding about the biochemical structure of certain foods and how they interact with the human digestive system. If this were not the case, then the human food industry would not market foods, such as nuts, soybeans, and certain vegetables, which are also eaten by animals.

Most creatures instinctively know the foods to eat, but humans are guided by intelligence; and any lack in it with respect to food brings us in harms way. Presently, humans eat just about anything. This has resulted in the epidemic of chronic disease, which is proof that a better understanding of nutrition is required.

Nutritionists have not considered the health consequences associated with eating foods that are anatomically designed for other creatures. Again, this is partly due to the fact that there is no national or international consensus among health experts about food distinctions with respect to foods that are meant for humans from those that are fit for other creatures. The Honorable Elijah Muhammad has brought this distinction to the forefront, but it has not been widely accepted. Only those few who have followed His advice have experienced excellent health, vitality, and youthfulness.

Medical scientists agree that diet is the foremost factor in the etiology of chronic diseases. As with the Honorable Elijah Muhammad, they also agree that overeating is the key factor that render enormous health complications. This, however, is where the agreement ceases.

Unlike this world's medical scientists, the Honorable Elijah Muhammad has set parameters for the frequency of food consumption. Neither the health studies presented in Chapter 2, nor the hundreds of others available, have addressed this most essential aspect. For example, He advises that humans eat, at a minimum, one meal every 24 hours—of the right foods. This, He has stated, is enough to sustain good health and foster longevity. *How important is this aspect in thwarting chronic diseases, particularly when overeating is the force behind the epidemic?* We must admit that it is very important, so how valid is any health study that does not consider this?

The Honorable Elijah Muhammad has also defined the right foods that humans should eat. In doing so, He does not assume that natural foods are good for humans simply because they are natural. He disagrees with the consumption of many natural foods that have been recommended by government health agencies and medical institutions. *If parameters are set for the frequency of food consumption, should not the best foods for human consumption also be isolated from the total pool of food?*

In settling this disagreement, the foremost question is: *How are bad or good foods distinguished?* The answer is relatively simple. Biological analyses that examines the biochemical structure of foods against the human digestive system is fundamental in determining whether or not the food in question is good for human consumption. Fortunately, biochemical and biological data is available and can be used to reach the necessary conclusions. In cases where this information is unavailable, experiments can be conducted to reach sound conclusions. However, as it stands, many natural foods have undergone biochemical analysis. In fact, biochemical analyses of natural foods have been engaged for more than a century. Nuts have been studied for many years, and information about their biochemical properties is readily available.

Biologically, the essential processes that sustain human life have long been identified. For example, the digestive system can only degrade the foods that meet the requirements of its physical and chemical capabilities. This is the foundation of the entire digestive process. So, despite the quantity of nutrients contained in foodstuffs, if they cannot be degraded by the digestive system, they have no place in the human diet.

Health studies that promote nut consumption, such as those conducted by major educational and medical institutions, neglect to mention or consider the biochemical data that, undoubtedly, show that nuts contain potent poisons that have long been determined harmful to humans. These poisons include protease inhibitors, lectins, phytates, goitrogens, and allergens.[38] The health impact of each of these poisons is addressed in the following sections.

Protease inhibitors

Description

Protease inhibitors are complex proteins that block the digestive action of enzymes that digest food proteins. They are found in many types of vegetation, particularly beans and nuts. Protease inhibitors are impermeable against proteases due to the integrity of their binding properties.

Protease inhibitors are known to be most potent when contained in foods that are in their raw stages. For example, eating raw beans brings a person in direct contact with these poisons. Biochemical studies have been conducted on the adverse impact of these poisons when present in both raw and processed foods.

In some studies, the protease inhibitors remained intact despite heat treatment. Protease inhibitors are thus classified as either heat-labile or heat-stable. Heat-labile protease inhibitors are proteins in which the complex bonds are effectively degraded by normal cooking. This makes them easy to digest, because the cooking process has done most of the work in preparing the food for digestion and absorption by the body.

Heat-stable protease inhibitors cannot be degraded by cooking or by protein digestive enzymes. They remain intact and, consequently, wreck havoc on the digestive system. Heat-stable protease inhibitors also permeate the intestinal lining, transforming themselves into potent allergens and other poisons.

Kunitz and Bowman-Birk are two classes of heat-stable protease inhibitors. They are known to contain disulfide bonds or bridges, which makes them stable against heat treatment and digestive enzymes. They are, particularly, known for their stability against trypsin and chymotrypsin, the two major protein-digesting enzymes in the body.

Impact on Body

The inhibitory activity of protease inhibitors has been studied for nearly a century. Most studies have confirmed that the greater adverse impact rendered by protease inhibitors has been against monogastric animals. Monogastric animals are those that possess only one stomach. Animals that possess multiple stomachs, such as birds, cattle, and sheep, were not adversely impacted by protease inhibitors.

The harm caused by protease inhibitors has been well documented. Their inhibitory activity registers two primary adverse health conditions: 1) body growth inhibition, and 2) pancreatic hypertrophy and hyperplasia, potentially leading to pancreatic cancer.

In the first condition, body growth inhibition, the impact of protease inhibitors must be understood in association with the importance of protein to the human body. Proteins have structural and metabolic roles, which are vital to all living organisms. Structurally, protein is the core building block of all cells. Metabolically, protein is responsible for catalyzing all the chemical reactions that take place within the cell. It converts chemical energy into mechanical energy, and is a building block for enzymes, hormones and antibodies.

The body growth inhibition caused by protease inhibitors results from the lack of adequate protein in the human body. The cells require protein to build bone and tissues. Therefore, a reduction in protein equates to a reduction in bone and tissue.

The second adverse impact, pancreatic hypertrophy, results when the pancreas continuously attempts to produce the enzymes required to degrade heat-stable protease inhibitors. This subject is further addressed in Chapter 7.

Found in Nuts

The presence of protease inhibitors in nuts has long been reported.[39] Nuts, especially peanuts, contain heat-stable protease inhibitors that block digestive enzymes.[40] Because they contain heat-stable protease inhibitors, honey-roasted peanuts and peanut butter products yet contain these poisons.

Those persons and health institutions that declare that peanuts are high in protein have failed to acknowledge that the protein content in peanuts is not readily digestible by humans. Therefore, it matters little whether nuts are high or low in protein, because only birds and creatures whose digestive systems are capable of degrading them are the benefactors of this high protein.

To date, the American Dietetic Association continues to tout a glass of milk and a peanut butter sandwich as a high protein meal for children. I recommend that the Association explore the biochemical research that proves otherwise, and rescind its deadly recommendation.

Lectins

Description

Lectins are complex proteins that have the unique property of binding to carbohydrate-containing molecules. These are usually molecules located on the surface of red blood cells. Thus, lectins cause red blood cells to clump together or agglutinate. This adverse action is, primarily, rendered against monogastric animals.

As with protease inhibitors, lectins are also widely distributed throughout the plant kingdom. They are most potent in raw vegetation; however, they continue to remain potent in some heat-treated vegetation.

Impact on Body

The health implications of lectins are monumental. Health detriments include:

- *the lowering of insulin levels in the blood;*
- *an inhibition of disaccharide-digesting proteases in the intestines;*
- *degenerative changes in the liver and kidneys; and*
- *interference with nonheme iron*

The most observable health implication registered by these poisons has been growth inhibition. However, given the adverse actions listed above, lectins are known to contribute to diabetes by lowering insulin levels in the blood. They also contribute to gastrointestinal tract disturbances by inhibiting proteases in the intestinal lining. Lectins also distress the liver and kidney, principally through their inhibition of carbohydrate digestion.

Found in Nuts

Lectins are, particularly, abundant in peanuts.[41-42] Biochemical analyses confirm that peanuts contain six major and three minor proteins capable of causing agglutination. Although moist heat treatment usually alleviates their presence, both raw and heat-processed peanuts are known to contain high levels of lectins.[43]

Again, those touting peanuts have failed to consider the presence of lectins and the potential harm they render to humans when ingested.

Phytates (Phytic Acid)

Description

Phytate or phytate acid is a cyclic compound that binds to metals such as calcium, magnesium, zinc, and iron, preventing the uptake and, subsequent use, of these minerals by the human body.[44-46] These compounds are often referred to as *metal* or *mineral binders*.

Impact on Body

The impact of phytates on the human body lies in the importance of minerals to the human body. Trace elements are essential to the body's homeostatic regulation, serving vital functions. For example, some trace elements—working in concert with proteins and other organic coenzymes—attract molecules and facilitate their conversion to specific end products that control vital biological functions.

Other trace elements either donate or accept electrons in reactions to reduction or oxidation, and thus, participate in the production of ATP. Some trace elements have a regulatory role. They control important biological processes through such actions as inhibiting enzymatic reactions; facilitating the binding of molecules to receptor sites on cell membranes; and inducing genes to form important molecules.

For example, iron binds to, transports, and releases oxygen in the body. It is among the most important trace elements and has been the subject of many studies, specifically, studies that analyze its interaction with metal-binding components in foods.[47]

Found in Nuts

Nuts are known to contain significant amounts of phytic acid and polyphenols. Nutritionally, phytic acid is contained in many vegetables; however, its adverse impact is only realized when the food that contains it also contains amounts of substances that counter its adverse reaction. One such substance is ascorbic acid (vitamin C).

For example, cauliflower, nuts, and soybeans contain significant levels of phytate acid. However, the binding action of phytates upon each of these foods is drastically different. The bioavailability of iron in cauliflower is very high because cauliflower contains a significant amount of abscorbic acid.

Contrarily, the bioavailability of iron is very low in diets that feature nuts and soybeans.[48] These foods contain little abscorbic acid; thus, the binding action of phytates on minerals is tremendous.

This aspect sheds light on the interrelationship of nutrients contained in food. This is also why research that focus on the so-called health benefits of one nutrient, alone, is inadequate. People usually don't eat a single nutrient. They eat food. In fact, most people eat meals that comprise various combinations of foods. The interaction of these molecules within the human body has a key role in the digestibility of that entire meal.

Unfortunately, little research is available about the interaction among different foods. The Honorable Elijah Muhammad recommends that we limit the types of foods that we consume at a single setting. He states that we do not need to eat a wide variety of foods—that two or three foods are sufficient to handle our nutritional needs.

In addition to the mineral-binding properties of phytates, other adverse impacts result from their consumption. Studies have shown phytates to, nonselectively, bind with proteins, inhibiting the action of digestive enzymes such as pepsin,[49] trypsin,[50-51] and amylase.[52-54] As with protease inhibitors, the obvious consequence is that protein is unavailable to foster growth.[55] This binding action also causes pancreatic distress.

Allergens

Description

Food allergens are food fragments responsible for allergic reactions. They are usually proteins within the food that are not broken down by the heat of cooking, stomach acids, or by the enzymes that digest proteins.

Impact on Body

Allergens cross the gastrointestinal lining, enter the bloodstream, and go to specific organs, causing allergic reactions throughout the body. These reactions range from mild discomforts to extremely severe health conditions, including death. This subject is taken up in greater detail in Chapter 11.

Found in Nuts

Nuts have long been known to contain allergens, and are generally regarded as a high allergenic food. In fact, the peanut is known for its notorious ability to cause severe and fatal allergic reactions.

Goitrogens

Description

Goitrogens are complex proteins, which bind with iodine, thus inhibiting the uptake of this mineral by the thyroid gland. This inhibitory action causes an inadequate production of thyroid hormones because iodine is one of two substances the thyroid uses to synthesize its vital hormones. Goitrogens are heat-stable, and therefore, remain intact despite various heat treatment methods.

Impact on Body

Goitrogens, ultimately, stress the thyroid gland, causing goiter. Goitrogens can cause malfunction in metabolism, which leads to an array of ailments and diseases. This subject is discussed in Chapter 8.

Found in Nuts

Peanuts, in particular, contain significant amounts of heat-stable goitrogens.[56] As such, peanuts are known to cause iodine deficiency. Some health publications have recommended that diets containing peanuts be supplemented with iodine. Unfortunately, such recommendations or warnings are absent from most bags of peanuts and peanut butter labels. Few people are aware that with each peanut they eat, their body is being robbed of dietary iodine.

CHAPTER 6

Endocrine System & Chronic Disease

Americans, as well as the human family in general, have long been under the burden of chronic diseases. More than 90 million Americans live with chronic illnesses, which also have, traditionally, accounted for the majority of all deaths. The major chronic diseases that lead to early mortality are cardiovascular diseases, cancer, and diabetes mellitus. In the U.S., these diseases account for approximately 70% of all causes of death, which translates into 1.7 million deaths annually.[57]

Chronic diseases also produce an astronomical financial toll of approximately a trillion dollars each year in health-related and loss productivity costs. According to the Centers for Disease Control and Prevention (CDC), the escalating health care costs that are accounting for an ever-increasing percentage of U.S. budget expenditures cannot be effectively addressed without first addressing the prevention of chronic diseases.

Chronic diseases are non-communicable and predominantly stem from improper dietary and lifestyle habits. This makes chronic diseases preventable and treatable through changes in dietary habits and lifestyle behaviors.

This chapter addresses the biological factors that give rise to chronic diseases, and describes those physiological mechanisms charged with maintaining the health of the body.

Disease Defined

Generally, the term "disease" can be defined as the disruption of vital biological processes that maintain the health of the body. Such disruptions render the body in a disoriented or imbalanced state. The severity of this imbalance determines the intensity and duration of the diseased state.

For example, a virus usually causes the common cold. The body recognizes the virus as foreign material and is prompted into action. This action is the engagement of various body mechanisms responsible for fending off the virus and restoring the body to its balanced state. These mechanisms, combined with rest and adequate fluid intake, are usually enough to remedy the common cold, and after several days to a week, the health of the body is restored. It re-enters the state of ease or wellness.

Chronic diseases, on the other hand, are acute, molecular disorders that disrupt the very mechanisms charged with maintaining balance within the body. Decades ago, the term used to describe these diseases was "degenerative". This term inferred that the body was in a drastic state of decline through cellular degeneration. This meant that the cells were no longer able to facilitate their life-sustaining processes, so the reversal was underway. As the cell's ability to sustain its life declines, so does the health of the person.

The term "chronic" was later installed to describe the tenacious and enduring characteristics of these diseases, without trivializing the life-threatening nature associated with them. According to the CDC, chronic diseases are *illnesses that are prolonged, do not resolve spontaneously, and are rarely cured completely*. They represent sustained collapses in mechanisms that support the human body.

This definition calls into question the validity of short-term health studies, which alleges results that appear favorable because of immediate changes in levels of biological fluids (.i.e LDL, HDL, and triglyceride levels). Again, not only are the results of such studies meager, but as previously stated, they have little sustainability.

Controlling Systems: Nervous & Endocrine

The foremost priority of all biological mechanisms is to keep the body in a state of balance. This means that the body's internal environment must be stable—a process that is referred to as *homeostasis.* Homeostasis means unchanging, and must be accomplished despite the continuous changes that occur inside and outside the body. Of course, changes continuously occur within the body, so the concept actually refers to the state of equilibrium or balance, in which internal conditions vary, but always within relatively narrow limits.

Homeostasis cannot take place unless the various systems and mechanisms that control the body are able to communicate with each other. Therefore, communication is the essential factor for homeostasis, and is accomplished by the body's two controlling and communication systems: the nervous and endocrine. Combined, these systems coordinate and direct all cellular activities.

The nervous system uses electrical impulses that produce immediate action so that rapid adjustments can be made in response to changes occurring inside and outside the body. The more slowly acting endocrine system uses chemical messengers that produce temporal responses, which are more prolonged.

Despite these differences, both systems are intrinsically integrated, at the hypothalamus. The hypothalamus is thus known as a neuroendocrine organ. Both systems also have important similarities. First, transmission of information from one cell to the other is via chemical messengers and, second, the target cells possess specific receptors for these chemical messengers.

Endocrine System: Organs and Hormones

The major endocrine organs are the pituitary, thyroid, parathyroid, adrenal, pineal, thymus, pancreas, and gonad glands. As previously discussed, the hypothalamus is considered a neuroendocrine organ because, in partnership with the pituitary gland, it plays a key role in regulating hormonal processes of all endocrine glands.

The pituitary gland hangs from the base of the brain and is enclosed by bone. Structurally, the gland consists of a hormone-producing glandular portion (anterior pituitary) and a neural portion (posterior), which is an extension of the hypothalamus. The pituitary gland is considered the master endocrine gland because it combines with the hypothalamus to control feedback mechanisms, and its hormones control the hormonal activity of other endocrine organs.

Neurons controlled by the hypothalamus monitor homeostasis, and the hypothalamus discharges hormones into the anterior-pituitary. When the anterior-pituitary receives this chemical stimulus from the hypothalamus, it releases its hormones. These hormones are of two major types: inhibiting and releasing.

The targeted organs or cells respond by synthesizing and secreting the proper hormones in response to specific releasing hormones, or by halting hormone release in response to inhibiting hormones. And, although many different releasing and inhibiting hormones pass from the hypothalamus to the anterior-pituitary, the individual target cells are able to distinguish the messages directed to them.

Hormones are known to have various roles, including acting as neurotransmitters; however, their core action is to alter cell activity by sustaining, increasing or decreasing the rates of normal cellular processes. A hormone stimulus typically produces one or more of the following:

- *changes in plasma membrane permeability and/or electrical state by opening or closing ion channels;*
- *synthesis of proteins or certain regulatory molecules, such as enzymes, within the cell;*
- *enzyme activation or deactivation;*
- *induction of secretory activity; and*
- *stimulation of mitosis.*

Figure 6. Endocrine System

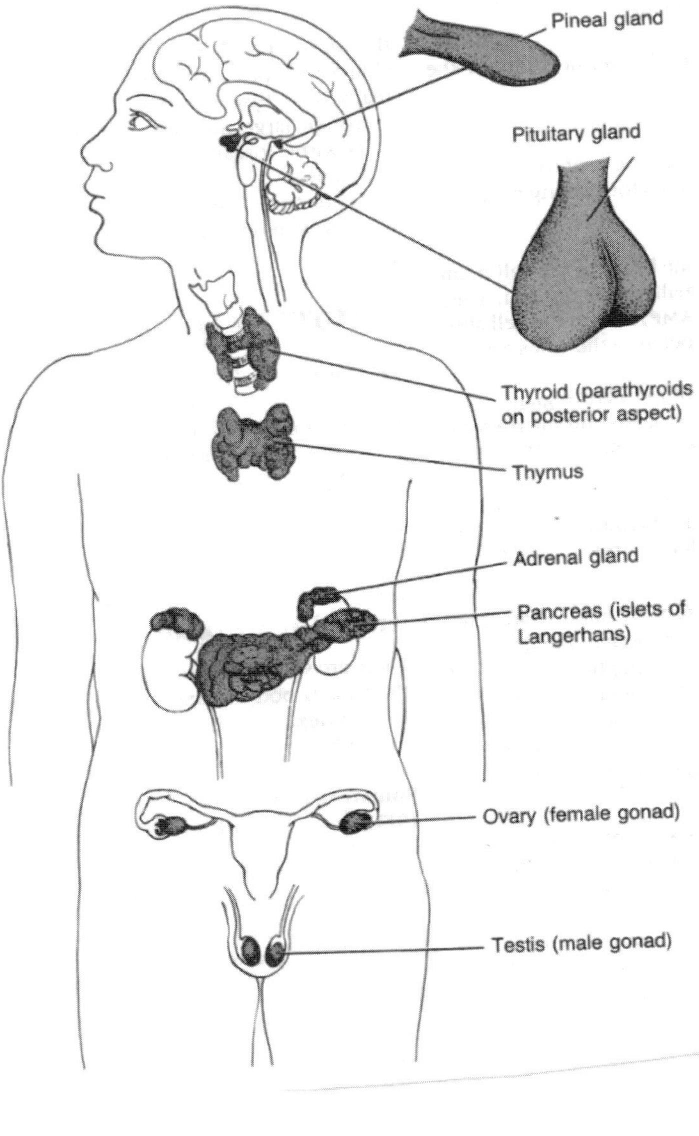

Hormonal regulated processes include reproduction; growth and development; mobilization of body defenses to stressors; maintenance of electrolyte, water, and nutrients balances; and regulation of cellular metabolism.

Endocrine's Biofeedback Mechanisms

As previously discussed, the health of the body is dependent upon homeostasis. The body is in homeostasis when its needs are adequately met and its functions are occurring smoothly. Every organ and body system has a role in maintaining the constancy of the internal environment.

Adequate blood levels of vital nutrients must be continuously present, and heart activity and blood pressure must be constantly monitored and adjusted so that the blood is propelled with adequate force to reach all body tissues. Also, wastes must not accumulate, and body temperature must be precisely controlled. Basically, a wide variety of chemical, thermal, and neural factors act and interact to maintain homeostasis.

The endocrine system is essential to homeostatic control, which has three principal components. The first component is a receptor, which is a sensor that monitors the environment and responds to changes by sending information to the second element, the control center. The flow of information from the receptor to the control center occurs along the third component—the afferent pathway. The control center, which determines the set point at which a variable is to be maintained, analyzes the input it receives and then determines the appropriate response. This process is also called the biofeedback mechanism.

An excellent example of the biofeedback mechanism is the handling of dietary glucose. It is essential for the body to regulate plasma glucose concentration. If the glucose concentration is too low, brain cell functions are impaired and coma occurs. If the plasma glucose is too high, glucose is lost in the urine, and high glucose also has toxic effects on the cells lining the walls of blood vessels.

When one eats a normal meal, the pancreas (the source of insulin) is informed by neural signals from both the head and the intestine.

These nerves release acetylcholine and cholecystokinin, respectively, and sensitize the pancreas' beta cells so that when the glucose is absorbed from the intestine and causes an increase in blood glucose concentration, the beta cells respond with an increase in the insulin secretion.

This effect of glucose is further enhanced by hormones such as cholecystokinin, gastric inhibitory peptide, and glucagon-like peptide-1, all of which act on the beta cell. Hence, an increase in blood glucose concentration causes a large change in the insulin secretory rate.

When insulin is secreted into the blood stream, glucose is taken up by most body cells, and the excess is stored as glycogen in the liver and muscles. The action of insulin brings blood sugar levels back to normal and the stimulus that promotes the release of insulin.

Disruption of Biofeedback Mechanism

The biofeedback mechanism is so important that most diseases, especially chronic diseases, usually result from its disruption. When this biofeedback system becomes disrupted, the body is endangered. In the case of glucose regulation, the biofeedback mechanism becomes inoperable when the pancreas is not able to produce the insulin required to manage the rising glucose levels. The result is diabetes, a metabolic disorder that produces a domino effect, as it disturbs other biofeedback mechanisms.

There is an interrelationship among all biofeedback mechanisms, so a disruption of one usually causes disruptions in others. This is why some diseases are also risk factors for other diseases. Diabetes is a risk factor for heart disease, which is also connected to a biofeedback mechanism, specifically the one that manages blood-lipid levels.

The body's ability to regulate its internal environment is essential for health. There are numerous biofeedback mechanisms at work in the body, and all have the primary goal of preventing sudden severe changes within the body. Some of these biofeedback mechanisms control body temperature, regulate heart rate, blood pressure, and blood levels of oxygen, carbon dioxide, and minerals.

The endocrine system regulates these continuous processes, which go on for relatively long periods of time. Dysfunctions in these processes are gradually manifested, sometimes over extended durations. Consequently, these dysfunctions result in diseases that usually require an extended amount of time to resolve.

Malfunctions in the endocrine system are at the root of most chronic diseases, and since these diseases are diet-related then endocrine malfunction is significantly linked to dietary practices.

The next two chapters show the means by which the poisons contained in nuts negatively impact the endocrine system, specifically the pancreas and thyroid glands. These poisons—protease inhibitors, goitrogens, lectins, and allergens—dismantle the body's homeostasis, causing an array of diseases to occur.

The Honorable Elijah Muhammad states that five years is taken from a person's lifespan every time he or she eat nuts. The assignment of this precise impact warrants the utmost consideration, and is addressed in the following chapters. We can surmise that these health implications have reduced the human life span to its current meager limit of 65 to 75 years, as nuts and other animal foods have been a mainstay in the human diet for centuries.

CHAPTER

7

Nut Protease Inhibitors and the Pancreas

The pancreas is one of the most important organs in the body. It serves as both a digestive and endocrine organ. Located behind the stomach, this triangular organ is composed of endocrine and exocrine gland cells.

The exocrine acinar cells produce the enzyme-rich digestive juices. These juices, comprised of enzymes, are ducted into the small intestines during food digestion, and are responsible for degrading proteins, fats, and starches—the major food molecules used by the cell for building blocks and energy.

The pancreas' endocrine cells, pancreatic islets (islets of Langerhans), produce pancreatic hormones, namely the glucagon-synthesizing alpha cells and the insulin-producing beta cells. Insulin and glucagon are involved in the regulation of blood glucose levels. Their effect on the blood glucose level is opposite, as insulin lowers blood-glucose and glucagon raises it.

The pancreas' islet cells also synthesize several other important substances. These include somatostatin, which inhibits the release of insulin and glucagon; and pancreatic polypeptide, which is secreted by the F cells. Pancreatic polypeptide has a role in regulating the organ's exocrine functions.

As stated in the previous chapter, protease inhibitors are proteins that are not degradable by protein-digesting enzymes. They have an affinity to these enzymes, and consequently, inhibit their catabolic actions. *What is the impact of protease inhibitors on the human body? How does the body respond to this poison?* Obviously, the response is not favorable, as poison is not favorable, but what precisely is the response?

Figure 7. Human Pancreas

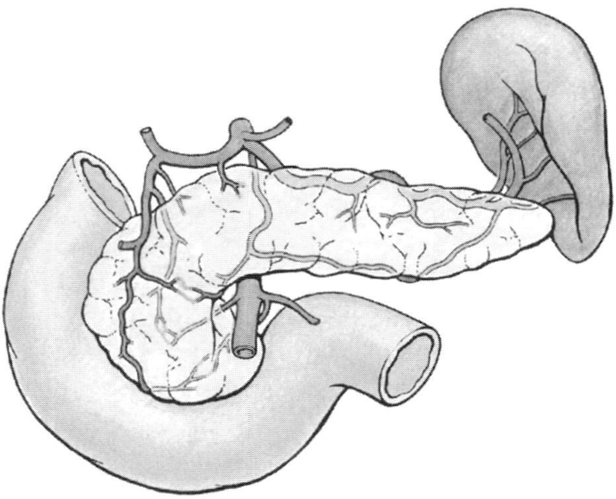

Fortunately, protease inhibitors have been one of the most widely researched naturally-occurring plant toxins. Hundreds of studies have been conducted on them, primarily because the importance of protein to the body warrants this attention. Most of these studies have been conducted with lower animals, and the effect of protease inhibitors has been well established.

Generally, the studies showed that monogastric animals experienced a significant lack of body growth.[58,59] This is an obvious response, since protein is the building blocks of body tissue.

The research showed that the animals were not benefiting from the protein, although they consumed "high protein" foods. It is also important to note that in some studies the animals eventually died of poisoning.[60,61] This reaffirms the fact that protein quality, and not quantity, is the most important factor that determines whether a protein food is of value to the eater.

The most significant physiological impact caused by the consumption of protease inhibitors was abnormal enlargement of the animals' pancreas.[63] Histologically, this enlargement was the result of pancreatic *hypertrophy* and *hyperplasia. Pancreatic hypertrophy* occurs when the pancreatic cells increase or swell beyond their normal size. *Pancreatic hyperplasia* occurs when there is an abnormal increase in the number of pancreatic cells.

The cause behind these adverse reactions was due to the pancreas' attempt to increase its secretion of digestive enzymes, particularly trypsin and chymotrypsin. This led researchers to conclude that the growth depression caused by protease inhibitors was not only caused by the unavailability of protein, but also was due to the loss of amino acids through enzymes that were being secreted by a hyperactive pancreas.[63,64]

Furthermore, some studies revealed that protease inhibitors had the potential to cause pancreatic cancer, which was an end result of hyperplasia. For example, the findings in one study showed an appearance of adenomatous nodules on the pancreas.[65]

Despite these studies, foods with heat-stable protease inhibitors are permitted on the market. This is due to the lack of integration between agricultural, medical, and nutritional entities and their respective research. Many are just unaware of such studies. However, because soybeans contain similar protease inhibitors, some consumer advocates have opposed the marketing of foods that contain potent protease inhibitors.

This has created controversy with respect to the vast marketing of soybean products. Scientists who represent food manufacturers have suggested that there has not been enough studies conducted on humans to determine whether or not our response to protease inhibitors is the same as that of lower animals.[66]

The question with regard to this position is how many studies are enough? There has been human studies conducted with plant protease inhibitors. In these studies, the human pancreas' reaction to protease inhibitors registered the same adverse effects as that documented in animal studies—hypersecretion of pancreatic juices.[67] The digestive enzymes, whether in animals or humans, cannot degrade heat-stable protease inhibitors. The pancreas operates the same, whether in animals or humans.

For example, the secretion of pancreatic juice is regulated by a biofeedback mechanism. Pancreatic enzyme secretion is inversely related to the levels of pancreatic juices in the small intestines. When protein-rich chyme enters the small intestines, the hormone, Cholecytokinin (CCK), is released from the intestinal walls. This hormone stimulates the pancreas to secrete digestive enzymes, namely, trypsin and chymotrypsin, into the small intestine. Once the pancreatic juice enters the small intestine and there is a reduction in the presence of protein molecules, CCK is triggered to "shut off".

Protease inhibitors, however, form enzyme-inhibitor complexes with the protein-digesting enzymes. The protein or protease inhibitor is never degraded, therefore its presence remains high. Consequently, CCK continues to stimulate pancreatic secretion.

The pancreas eventually becomes overworked. The pancreas, responding to CCK's continuous call, swells as it attempts to produce more pancreatic juice. This swelling is due to pancreatic hypertrophy and hyperplasia.

Disruption of Digestive Function

The primary substances that drive the chemical digestive process are bile, which is produced by the liver, and pancreatic digestive juices. Pancreatic digestive juices contain four major categories of digestive enzymes: amylase, which degrades starch into sugar; trypsin and chymotrypsin, which are proteolytic (protein-splitting) enzymes; lipase, which splits fats; and rennin, a milk-curdling enzyme.

These pancreatic enzymes have the responsibility of digesting foods; therefore, poisons that either hinder or impair the pancreas, compromises the timely delivery of essential digestive juices to the small intestines. The result is that the ability to digest food and absorb its nutrients is impaired or halted. The end result is sickness, disease, and ultimately death.

Protease inhibitors impair the pancreas, and consequently, disrupt the digestive process, causing three critical events:

- *protein is unavailable, leading to malnutrition;*
- *there is a mobilization and, subsequent exhaustion, of endogenous amino acids; and*
- *pancreatic hypertrophy and hyperplasia result, causing the pancreas to malfunction*

In the first event, protein is unavailable because the protein, itself, is comprised of protease inhibitors. Without protein, the cell is not able to facilitate its life-sustaining functions. As the cell weakens and die, body tissues and organs weaken. There is a degeneration of body tissue and organs, which is at the root of the many chronic diseases.

In the second event, the biological conditions that result from the absence of dietary protein is intensified. Since pancreatic enzymes, such as trypsin and chymotrypsin, are comprised of amino acids (as all enzymes are), the effect of a hyperactive pancreas diverts these amino acids from the synthesis of body tissue protein to the synthesis of enzymes. These enzymes are dispatched into the small intestines where they, too, are inhibited by the protease inhibitors.

The obvious effect of these activities is a loss of tissue mass due to the exacerbation of an already critical situation—wherein food protein is unavailable to the body because the food is comprised of indigestible proteins.

The third event that occurs as a result of ingesting protease inhibitors is pancreatic swelling—hypertrophy and hyperplasia. As previously noted, these conditions result from a severely distressed pancreas. The pancreas is furiously attempting to generate digestive juices in order to maintain homeostasis. It eventually swells or enlarges, as an attempt to convert amino acids into digestive enzymes. As a final resort, the pancreas produces additional islets, which leads to hyperplasia.

The biological logic is that more cells will produce more enzymes. This logic is similar to the logic wherein the body produces more adipose cells to accommodate excess nutrients. As with the process of obesity, this process is not instant, but gradually occurs over a duration, as most people consume nuts and other foods containing protease inhibitors throughout their lifetimes. The pancreas gradually fails causing a host of other health conditions.

According to the biological underpinnings of the digestive process, the inactivation of, or insufficiency in the production of proteolytic enzymes also increases the risk that protein molecules will be absorbed in their undigested forms. This provokes inflammatory reactions at distant tissues and organs. And, if at the same time the circulating anti-inflammatory enzymes are deficient, as a further consequence of pancreatic exhaustion, then the ability of the body to deal with such inflammatory reactions (allergic or otherwise) is reduced or absent, culminating in arthritis.

When inadequate breakdown of ingested protein occurs and amino acid deficiency results—despite high intakes of food protein—the consequences usually include the difficulty, or inability, on the part of the body to produce adequate enzymes, hormones, and antibodies. This causes excessive demands to be made on a wide range of minerals and vitamins, particularly zinc and magnesium, which leads to deficiencies in these essential elements. And, because essential minerals are among the core molecules driving the immune system, the ability to adequately defend the body under these conditions is severely compromised.

Furthermore, as the pancreas degenerates, it becomes subjected to acute or chronic inflammation, atrophy, tumors, fatty necrosis, cysts, sclerosis, and abscesses. Acute pancreatitis may also result. And, as stated, the insufficient secretion of insulin causes diabetes mellitus.

These conditions usually start to occur between the ages of 30 and 40 years. This is why anyone over 40 years of age is at risk of diabetes. This, alone, proves that a gradual degeneration of the pancreas is taking place. This makes the consumption of protease inhibitors a root cause of diabetes.

Disruption of Endocrine Function

A malfunctioning pancreas compromises the production and provision of vital hormones, namely glucagon, insulin, somatostatin, and pancreatic polypeptide. When these substances are inadequately produced, the adverse results are phenomenal and lead to long-term chronic disorders. Following is a brief description of the roles of glucagon and insulin.

Glucagon

Glucagon is an extremely potent hyperglycemic hormone, as a single molecule of it can cause approximately 100 million molecules of glucose to be released into the blood stream. Glucagon facilitates three important activities:

- *it breaks down glycogen to glucose (glycogenolysis);*
- *it synthesizes glucose from lactic acid and from noncarbohydrate molecules, such as fatty acids and amino acids; and*
- *it causes the release of glucose by the liver cells into the blood, which causes blood sugar levels to rise.*

A secondary effect caused by the release of glucagon is a fall in the concentration of amino acids in the blood as the liver cells gather them to make new glucose molecules.

Secretion of glucagon is prompted by declining blood sugar levels. Conversely, glucagon release is suppressed by rising blood sugar levels and by the release of somatostatin. And, because glucagon is such an important hyperglycemic agent, it has been speculated that people with persistently low blood sugar levels (hypoglycemics) are deficient of this hormone.

Insulin

Insulin's main effect is to lower blood sugar levels. It does this by enhancing membrane transport of glucose (and other simple sugars) into body cells, especially muscle cells. Insulin also inhibits the breakdown of glucagon to glucose.

After glucose enters the target cells, insulin binds to glucose and triggers the following enzymatic activities:

- *catalyzes the oxidation of glucose for adenosine 5′-triphospate (ATP) production (ATP is the most important form of chemical energy in most cells);*
- *joins glucose together to form glycogen, and*
- *converts glucose to fat (in adipose tissue).*

The activities of insulin are prioritized, and as such, the energy needs of the body are met first, then glycogen is formed and deposited in the muscles. Finally, any excess glucose is converted to fat, which is then stored in fat cells.

Insulin also induces amino acid uptake and protein synthesis in muscle tissue. So, although elevated blood sugar levels is the chief stimulant of insulin secretion, rising plasma levels of amino acids and fatty acids also trigger insulin release.

Therefore, insulin also influences protein and fat metabolism. It inhibits the conversion of amino acids and fatty acids to glucose; thus, it counters any metabolic activity that would increase plasma levels of glucose. As the cells take up sugar and other nutrients, and plasma levels of these substances drop, insulin secretion is shut off.

Other hormones also, directly and indirectly, influence insulin release. For example, any hyperglycemic hormone, such as glucagon, called into action as blood sugar levels drop, indirectly stimulates insulin release by promoting glucose entry into the bloodstream.

As noted, somatostatin depresses insulin release, thus, blood sugar levels ultimately reflect a balance of both humoral and hormonal influences. Insulin and (indirectly) somatostatin are hypoglycemic factors that counter and counterbalance the hyperglycemic hormones.

Figure 8. Blood glucose regulation

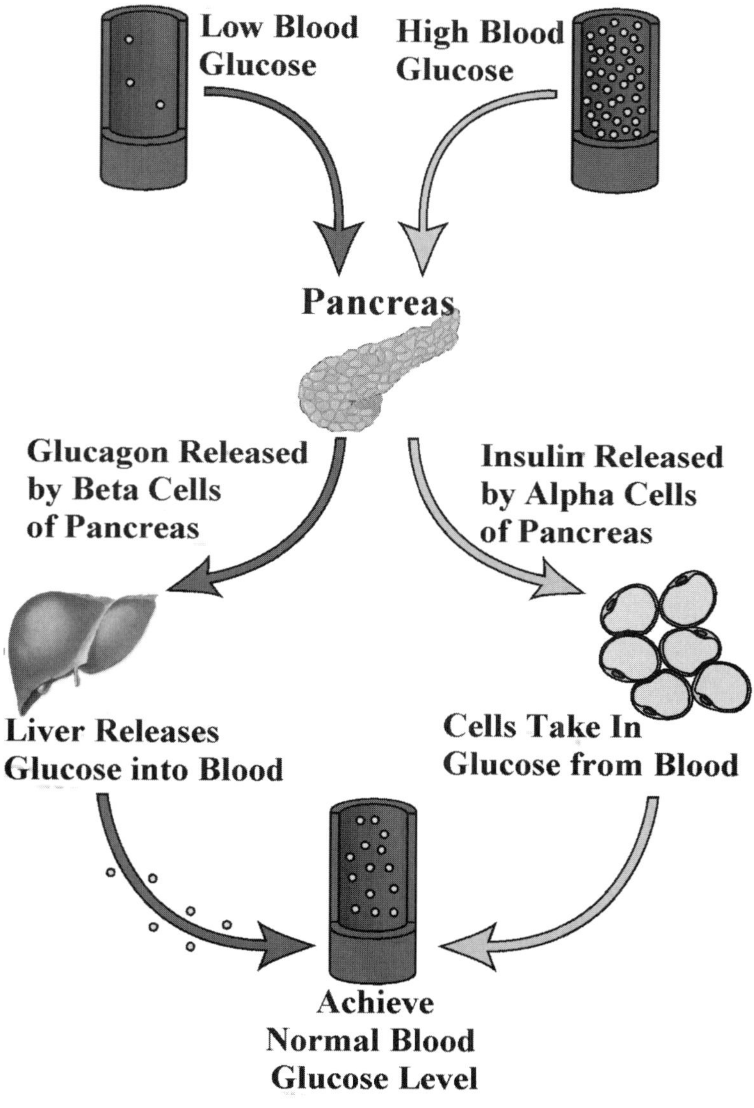

The critical role that both hormones—glucagon and insulin—play in ensuring the health of the human body has been described. When these hormones are deficient, the risks for chronic diseases increase.

As noted, insulin also has a critical role in managing ingested protein and fat. This particular aspect bears heavily on the fact that the overeating of all foods—fats, protein, and starches—not only causes the pancreas to expend its digestive juices, but also its insulin stores.

Common Diseases of Pancreas Malfunction

It is generally known that insufficient insulin production causes the dreaded disease, diabetes mellitus. We have also discussed pancreas malfunction as a probable cause of arthritis. These two diseases are examined in greater detail in the following sections.

Diabetes mellitus

The enormous detrimental impact rendered by protease inhibitors on the pancreas, at the very least, is responsible for the debilitating disease, diabetes mellitus. According to the Expert Committee on the Diagnosis and Classification of Diabetes Mellitus,[68] diabetes mellitus is a group of metabolic diseases characterized by hyperglycemia, which results from defects in insulin secretion, insulin action on cells, or both.

The vast majority of cases of diabetes fall into two broad categories: type 1 and type 2. Type 1 is an autoimmune dysfunction that causes the immune system to destroy the insulin-producing beta-cells of the pancreas. The more prevalent form of diabetes, type 2, is caused by a combination of factors, namely the cell's resistance to insulin and an inadequate secretion of insulin by the pancreas.

Diabetes is associated with long-term damage, dysfunction, and failure of various organs, especially the eyes, kidneys, nerves, heart, and blood vessels. Diabetes registers three notable symptoms: polyuria, polydipsia, and polyphagia.

The excessive glucose in the kidney filtrate acts as an osmotic diuretic, inhibiting water resorption by the kidney tubules. This causes polyuria—a huge urine output that leads to decreased blood volume and dehydration. Many electrolytes are also loss to polyuria, causing mineral imbalance.

The electrolyte imbalance caused by polyuria causes the person to get abdominal pains and vomit. This causes dehydration, which stimulates hypothalamic thirst centers, causing polydipsia, or excessive thirst. Additionally, there is an excessively abnormal hunger for food, which is called "polyphagia".

Polyphagia is caused by the absence of satiety that is usually experienced when glucose enters the cells. The diabetic must overcome strong cravings that are metabolically induced.

Acute, life-threatening consequences of diabetes may also occur. Diabetic mortality usually results from hyperglycemia with ketoacidosis. Pathologically, when sugars cannot be used as cellular fuel, more fats are mobilized, resulting in high fatty acid levels in the blood, a condition commonly referred to as lipidemia. Additionally, a decrease in plasma insulin concentration brings about the release of fatty acids from adipose tissue.

In severe cases of diabetes mellitus, blood levels of fatty acids and their metabolites, namely acetoacetic acid and acetone, rise dramatically. The fatty acid metabolites, collectively called ketones or ketone bodies, are strong organic acids. When they accumulate faster than they can be used or excreted, the blood pH drops, resulting in ketoacidosis, and ketones begin to spill into the urine (ketonuria).

The nervous system responds to these life-threatening conditions by initiating rapid deep breathing to blow off carbon dioxide from the blood and increase blood pH. If untreated, ketoacidosis disrupts virtually all physiological processes, including heart activity and oxygen transport. It can prompt severe depression of the nervous system, which can lead to comatosis and, finally, death.

Significant losses of body electrolytes also occur because of the need to rid the body of excess ketones. Because ketones are negatively charged, they carry out with them positive ions, specifically sodium and potassium. Mechanisms that depend on these vital minerals are also disrupted.

For example, both minerals—sodium and potassium—are responsible for maintaining proper fluid balance within the body's cells. Potassium controls more of the cells' internal fluids, while sodium controls more of the surrounding or external fluid of the cell.

Potassium is considered one of the most important minerals because it performs several vital functions, which include:

- *transporting electrical energy that nurtures and activates muscles and organs;*
- *regulating heart muscle action and arterial blood pressure;*
- *helping to facilitate enzyme reactions throughout the body;*
- *regulating blood pH and participating in the formation of Glycogen in the liver, muscles, and cartilage; and*
- *helping the kidneys eliminate waste matter, therefore assisting in eliminating blood impurities.*

Furthermore, potassium feeds the entire endocrine system, and thus aids in the increase of glandular secretions. This means that the endocrine system, at large, is significantly impacted by the loss of potassium.

Sodium, likewise, has critical responsibilities. These include:

- *making blood minerals soluble;*
- *aiding the formation of saliva and other digestive enzymes, while maintaining the correct amount of water in the body;*
- *neutralizing acidity in the blood;*
- *aiding the lymphatic system; and*
- *preventing the over-coagulation of the blood, thus protecting against blood clots in the brain and elsewhere.*

Sodium is required for proper muscle contraction. Sodium is also necessary to hold the body's calcium and magnesium in solution.

Potassium and sodium levels determine the body's strength and its ability to adapt to climate and weather changes. These two minerals must be in correct balance for the body to function normally.

People with diabetes also have an increased incidence of atherosclerotic cardiovascular, peripheral vascular, and cerebrovascular diseases. Hypertension, abnormalities of lipoprotein metabolism, and periodontal disease often result. These extreme metabolic disruptions also lead to long-term complications, which include:

- *retinopathy with potential loss of vision;*
- *nephropathy, leading to renal failure;*
- *peripheral neuropathy with risk of foot ulcers, amputations, and Charcot joints; and*
- *autonomic neuropathy causing gastrointestinal, genitourinary, and cardiovascular and sexual dysfunction.*

When considering the tremendous health detriments associated with diabetes, foods that contain these heat stable toxins should be banned from the market. Eating nuts is not worth this enormous price.

Arthritis

Arthritis, as previously described, is another disease that is linked to the consumption of protease inhibitors. The term, "arthritis," categorizes the diseases and conditions that affect the joints, the surrounding tissues, and other connective tissues. A few of these conditions include osteoarthritis, rheumatoid arthritis, lupus, gout, and fibromylgia.

The most common forms of arthritis are osteoarthritis and rheumatoid arthritis. Osteoarthritis is often termed "degenerative" or "age-related" joint disease, and most often affects the hip, knee, foot, and hand. Degeneration of joint cartilage and changes in underlying bone and supporting tissues lead to pain, stiffness, movement problems, and activity limitations.

Rheumatoid arthritis (RA), on the other hand, is characterized by chronic inflammation of the joint lining. Symptoms include pain, stiffness, and swelling of multiple joints. The inflammation may extend to other joint tissues and cause bone and cartilage erosion, joint deformities, movement problems, and activity limitations.

This condition can also affect connective tissue and blood vessels throughout the body, triggering inflammation in a variety of organs, including the lungs and heart. This increases a person's risk of dying of respiratory and infectious diseases.

According to current research on RA, there is an ongoing debate about the factors that contribute to the disease. No single or definitive cause has been attached to the disease. As a result, arthritis treatments range from medicated ointments and lotions, to pills and potions. There are, however, three etiological factors that most medical scientists agree contributes to RA.

One of these is that RA is caused by a bacteria infection. The second factor is that RA is caused by altered intestinal permeability, which causes food constituents and microbial components to penetrate the intestines. This leads to inflammation at distant sites, especially the joints.[69]

The third cause of arthritis is aging. As people get older, their joints and connective tissues degenerate. This reason, however, is not logically acceptable because aging is not clearly defined. Biologically, aging is simply cellular degeneration. Such degeneration is caused by factors that halt the cell's ability to reproduce and sustain itself.

Among the three causes given, health experts know that altered intestinal permeability is a leading cause of RA because polyarthritis is a common occurrence in intestinal disorders, specifically ulcerative colitis and Crohn's disease. Altered intestinal permeability refers to a condition wherein antigens, which normally would not penetrate the intestinal lining, are able to do so, primarily because the intestinal lining is damaged or weakened. *How does the intestinal mucosa or lining weaken?*

According to the Honorable Elijah Muhammad, the constant consumption of food gradually wears away the digestive organs. They become weakened and their ability to perform declines, producing numerous health ailments. The small intestine is constantly at work when food is eaten numerous times during the day. Eating three, four, and five meals a day keeps the small intestine, and other digestive organs in continuous labor. When this dietary practice goes on year-after-year, the organs weaken.

When a weakened small intestine is continuously penetrated by antigens, not only does arthritis occur, but its intensity increases with age. In addition, food allergies increase. Allergies that some people have never had to contend with are gradually acquired.

Rheumatoid arthritis is exacerbated by the ingestion of abrasive foods, such as nuts. This fact is validated in the treatment of some intestinal conditions. For example, in cases where people suffer from intestinal disorders, they are usually advised to refrain from eating nuts. Nuts are very hard on the digestive system, and usually pass through the digestive tract intact.

Furthermore, nut proteins, such as allergens, are known to permeate the intestinal lining, causing allergic reactions. Such permeability must be considered a significant risk factor for arthritis. In fact, arthritis also can be considered a chronic allergic reaction.

Altered intestinal permeability as a central cause of arthritis has also been validated through studies that show that fasting cures are the most effective remedies for treating RA. Several human studies have shown that fasting (going without food for one or more days) allows the body time to rest. This allows the body time to heal. This healing results in the strengthening of the small intestine.[70] The result is that the small intestine is not easily permeated, and antigens, which once passed freely, are unable to do so.[71]

In a study that featured a 10-day fast, it was reported that patients with RA had begun to feel better by the fifth day of fasting, and thus reported a reduction in stiffness and pain.[69] Additionally, all clinical tests that measured disease activity, showed remarkable reductions.

As a result of these studies, some countries are using fasting as a preferred treatment for RA and other diseases. Of course, America is not one of those places, as the commercial health care and pharmaceutical industries have promoted toxic drugs as leading remedies.

Both diabetes and arthritis are associated with endocrinological malfunctions that result from the consumption of protease inhibitors. The health of the pancreas and small intestine is of the utmost importance, and foods, such as nuts, viciously assault both organs, causing a myriad of problems.

Prevalence of Diseases Associated with Protease Inhibitors

Now that we have discussed the diseases associated with protease inhibitors, let us now turn our attention to the prevalence of these diseases in the United States, a land where nuts are both popular snacks and food ingredients.

Diabetes Mellitus

According to the National Institute of Diabetes, and Digestive and Kidney Diseases, more than 10 million Americans have been diagnosed with diabetes - 5.9% of the population - and more than half as many (5.4 million) may have the disease but do not know it.[72] Researchers have declared these figures to be underestimated. Nevertheless, diabetes has been officially designated as an epidemic.

Diabetes and its complications occur among Americans of all ages, racial and ethnic groups. The burden of this disease is more prevalent among elderly Americans, with more than 18% of adults over age 65 having diabetes. Diabetes is also significantly high among certain racial and ethnic populations, including African Americans, Hispanics/Latinos, and American Indians and Alaska Natives.

Diabetes is the leading cause of the following:

- *blindness in adults aged 20-74 years;*
- *end-stage (chronic and irreversible) kidney disease;*
- *lower-extremity amputations not related to injury.*

And, as stated, diabetes is a leading risk factor for heart disease, as people with diabetes are 2-4 times more likely to develop heart disease or stroke than people without diabetes.

The financial toll rendered by this disease is also phenomenal. The American Diabetes Association estimates that the nation spends more than $98 billion annually on both direct and indirect costs of diabetes.

Arthritis

Arthritis and other rheumatic conditions are among the most common chronic diseases. According to the CDC, these health conditions affect nearly 43 million Americans, or about one of every six people, making it one of the most prevalent diseases in the country.[73] Arthritis is also the leading cause of disability in the United States. It limits the everyday activities of more than 7 million Americans.

Each year, arthritis results in 44 million outpatient visits and almost three-quarters of a million hospitalizations. Estimated medical care costs for people with arthritis is $15 billion annually, and total costs (medical care and lost productivity) is estimated at almost $65 billion annually.

The impact of arthritis is expected to increase dramatically as "baby boomers" age. By 2020, an estimated 60 million Americans, or almost 20% of the population, will be affected by arthritis, and nearly 12 million will experience activity limitations. As with the prevalence of arthritis, the prevalence of arthritis-related disability is also expected to rise by the year 2020, when an estimated 11.6 million people will be affected. Thus, arthritis has become one of the most pressing public health problems—a problem that is expected to worsen unless prompt and responsible action is taken. Unfortunately, the promotion of nuts is not one of these actions. Contrarily, nut-promotion ensures that this dreaded forecast becomes a reality.

CHAPTER 8

Nut Goitrogens and the Thyroid Gland

The thyroid is a butterfly shaped gland, which wraps around the front part of the windpipe, located just below the Adam's apple. It is the largest endocrine organ in the human body, and is a component of an integrated organ complex known as the hypothalamic-pituitary-thyroid axis. This ductless gland traps and organifies the trace dietary element, iodine, which it uses to produce thyroid hormones.

The importance of the thyroid gland to the human body lies in the importance of its hormones: thyroxine and triiodothyronine. Thyroxine is the major hormone secreted by the thyroid gland, while most triiodothyronine is formed at the target tissues by conversion of thyroxine to triiodothyronine. Both hormones are similar, as each is constructed from two tyrosine amino acids. The difference between them is that thyroxine has four iodine atoms bound to it, while triiodothyronine has three.

Thyroid hormones affect nearly every cell in the body. Their dominant role is in cellular metabolism. For example, thyroid hormones stimulate enzymes concerned with glucose oxidation, and as such, control basal metabolic rate and body heat production. Thyroid hormones also cause an increase in the number of adrenergic receptors in blood vessels, so they play an important role in maintaining blood pressure.

Generally, these hormones affect heart rate, cholesterol level, body weight, energy level, muscle strength, skin condition, menstrual regularity, and memory. The hormones are also an important regulator of tissue growth and development, especially in the skeletal, nervous and reproductive systems. Table 2 lists the vital functions performed by the thyroid hormones.

Figure 9. Human Thyroid Gland

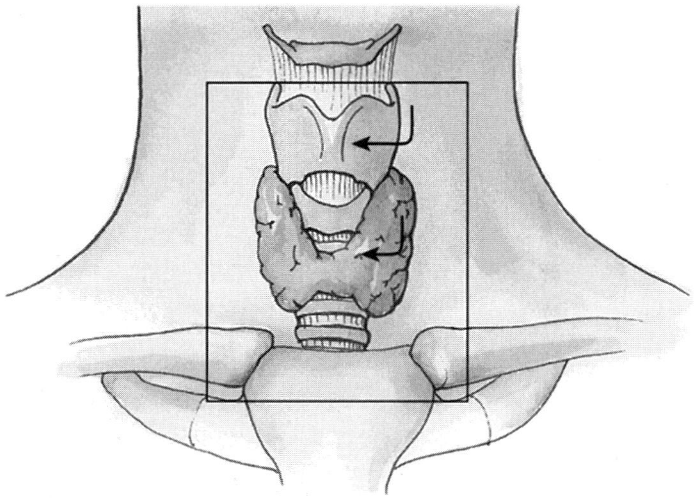

Thyroid Biofeedback Mechanism

As previously stated, endocrinological processes are facilitated through biofeedback mechanisms. Thyroid-releasing hormone (TRH) secreted by the hypothalamus acts on thyrotrophs in the anterior pituitary gland to stimulate the secretion of thyroid-stimulating hormone (TSH). TSH acts on the acinar cells of the thyroid gland to stimulate the release of thyroxine. The resulting increase in plasma thyroxine concentrations acts as a biofeedback signal on TRH-secreting cells in the hypothalamus and on the thyrotrophs in the anterior pituitary to inhibit TSH secretion.

TSH regulates and stimulates the active transport of inorganic iodide from the blood into the thyroid gland. Once inside the thyroid cells, iodide is oxidized to iodine. It is then combined with tyrosine to form thyroxine.

Figure 10. Thyroid hormones production

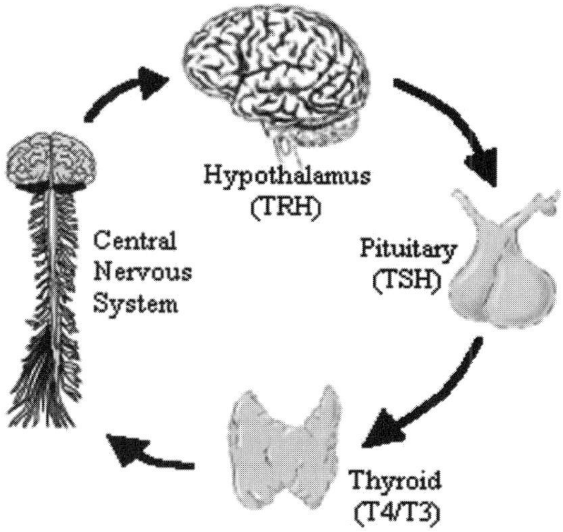

When dietary iodine is adequate, thyroid hormone is produced in normal amounts, particularly at a low level of TSH. Contrarily, when dietary iodine is limited, TSH secretion is increased, and the uptake of iodine by the thyroid is intensely promoted.

The thyroid gland, if operating adequately, stores enough thyroid hormone to last several months in the event that dietary iodine is not available. The total amount of iodine in the body is about 10-50 mg for an adult, and most of this is concentrated in the thyroid gland as thyroglobulin, a glycoprotein.

When the body needs stored thyroid hormones, proteolytic enzymes release them from thyroglobulin. Once released, the hormones then diffuse into the blood stream, where they are taken up by the cells. Once inside the cells, they influence cellular mechanisms, which in turn, influences every organ in the body.

Table 2. Major Effects of Thyroid Hormone in the Body

Process or System Affected	Normal Physiological Effects	Effects of Hyposecretion	Effects of Hypersecretion
Basal metabolic rate (BMR)/ temperature regulations	Promotes normal oxygen consumption and BMR; calorigenesis; enhances effects of catecholamines (and sympathetic nervous system)	BMR below normal; decreased body temperature; cold intolerance; decreased appetite; weight gain; decreased sensitivity to catecholamines	BMR above normal; increased body temperature; heat intolerance; increased appetite; weight loss; increased sensitivity to catecholamines may lead to high blood pressure
Carbohydrate/lipid/protein metabolism	Promotes glucose catabolism; mobilizes fats; essential for protein synthesis; enhances liver secretion of cholesterol	Decreased glucose metabolism; elevated cholesterol/triglyceride levels in blood; decreased protein synthesis; edema	Enhanced catabolism of glucose and fats; weight loss; increased protein catabolism; loss of muscle mass
Nervous system	Promotes normal development of nervous system in fetus and infant; necessary for normal adult system function	In infant, slowed/ deficient brain development, retardation; in adult, mental dulling, depression, paresthesias, memory impairment, listlessness, hypoactive reflexes	Irritability, restlessness, insomnia, over-responsiveness to environmental stimuli, exophthalmos, personality changes

Human Anatomy and Physiology. 3rd ed. 1995, New York, NY: The Benjamin/Cummings Publishing Company, Inc.

Table 2. Major Effects of Thyroid Hormone in the Body

Process or System Affected	Normal Physiological Effects	Effects of Hyposecretion	Effects of Hypersecretion
Cardiovascular system	Promotes normal functioning of the heart	Decreased efficiency of pumping action of the heart; low heart rate and blood pressure	Rapid heart rate and possible palpitating; high blood pressure; if prolonged, heart failure
Muscular system	Promotes normal muscular development, tone, and function	Sluggish muscle action; muscle cramps; myalgia	Muscle atrophy and weakness
Skeletal system	Promotes normal growth and maturation of the skeleton	In child, growth retardation, skeletal stunting/ malproportion, retention of child's body in adult, joint pain	In child, excessive skeletal growth initially, followed by early epiphyseal closure and short stature; in adult demineralization of skeleton
Gastrointestinal system	Promotes normal GI motility and tone; increases secretion of digestive juices	Depressed GI motility, tone, and secretory activity; constipation	Excessive GI motility; diarrhea; loss of appetite
Reproductive system	Promotes normal female reproductive ability and normal lactation	Depressed ovarian function; sterility; depressed lactation	In females, depressed ovarian function; in males, impotence
Integumentary system	Promotes normal hydration and secretory activity of skin	Skin pale, thickened, and dry; facial edema; hair coarse and thin; nails hard and thick	Skin flushed, thin, and moist; hair fine and soft; nails soft and thin

Human Anatomy and Physiology. 3rd ed. 1995, New York, NY: The Benjamin/Cummings Publishing Company, Inc.

Impact of Peanut Goitrogens on Thyroid Gland

As described in Chapter 4, goitrogens are naturally-occurring toxins that, when ingested by humans, bind with iodine, preventing its uptake and use by the thyroid gland. When iodine is unavailable because of goitrogenic activity, the body becomes deficient of iodine. The result is thyroid impairment, which leads to an array of major illnesses. Iodine deficiency is regarded as a critical health threat.

Iodine deficiency

Because iodine is required in the metabolism of virtually all cells, it plays an essential role in body growth and development. When the iodine level in the blood is low, the cells of the thyroid gland enlarge as an attempt to capture more iodine. This is similar to pancreatic hypertrophy caused by nut protease inhibitors.

Again, the mechanism behind this is the biofeedback mechanism that causes an increase in TSH levels. The low blood levels of thyroxine, which occur in iodine deficiency, stimulates the pituitary to produce TSH, which in turn stimulates the thyroid gland to work harder in order to produce thyroxine. This chronic adaptive condition causes abnormal growth of the gland or goiter. Goiter is a manifestation of iodine deficiency.

Goiters range in size from modest enlargements, to those that are several times the normal size. They are frequently nodular in appearance. Large goiters may cause obstruction of the trachea and esophagus, interfering with breathing and speaking. Although goiter is an observable sign of iodine deficiency, a person need not have a goiter to be iodine deficient.

There are several health disorders directly connected to iodine deficiency. These diseases are termed "iodine deficiency disorders" (IDD) and refer to the effects of iodine deficiency on the thyroid gland and overall health.

When the thyroid gland is not working properly, it can lead to a variety of long-term complications. Thyroid disorders can affect a person's cardiovascular and reproductive systems, and other major organs. Although there are several major thyroid diseases, the more common among them result from an underactive thyroid gland, or hypothyroidism. Hyperthyroidism, a condition wherein the thyroid produces more thyroid hormone than is needed, occurs less frequently.

There are numerous symptoms of hypothyroidism. A most common symptom is fatigue or lack of energy. Other physiological signs of prolonged hypothyroidism include: decreased metabolic rate, cold intolerance, weight gain, puffy face, dry skin, hoarse voice, edema, easy bruising, drooping upper eyelids, mental apathy, and problems with coordination. The more severe results of iodine deficiency, leading to thyroid health disorders, include sterility, osteoporosis, body deformation, thyroid cancer, high blood cholesterol and heart disease, and malfunctions of the circulatory and lymphatic systems.

Proof of Iodine Deficiency

In the United States, rises have been noted in both iodine deficiency and thyroid disease. In 1998, a study that was based upon the Centers for Disease Control and Prevention (CDC) National Health and Nutrition Examination Surveys (NHANES III 1988-1994), revealed that approximately 12 percent of Americans had low urine iodine concentrations (UI).[74] The study, *"Iodine Nutrition in the United States: Trends and Implications"* showed that urine iodine concentrations had decreased by more than half since the 1971-1974 NHANES I. The drop was dramatic—from 32 to 14.5 micrograms per deciliter (ug/dL).

According to the World Health Organization, UI concentrations in iodine-sufficient populations should be greater than 10 ug/dL, and no more than 20% of the populations should have UI concentrations less than 5 ug/dL. Although median UI concentrations from both NHANES 1 and NHANES II indicated adequate iodine intake for the overall U.S. populations, the median concentration decreased by more than 50% between the NHANES III and I.

The report indicated that the percentage of people excreting low concentrations of iodine had increased in all age groups. Most alarming, however, is a decrease in iodine concentrations among women. According to the report, approximately 6.7% of pregnant women, and 14.9% of women of childbearing age had UI concentrations below 5 ug/dL. Additionally, women 40-49 and 50-59 years of age, and other women of childbearing age were at-risk of low iodine concentrations. This references the increasing prevalence of thyroid problems and depressive disorders among women.[75]

Because iodine deficiency in fetuses and infants can lead to irreversible intellectual deficits,[76] the increasing proportion of women of child-bearing age and pregnant women who are in iodine deficiency range concerns health researchers. The major concern of iodine deficiency with respect to this study is not the numerous health implications associated with thyroid dysfunction, but the fact that iodine deficiency is the leading cause of mental retardation. Numerous studies have been conducted to validate the association of prolonged iodine deficiency to learning disabilities, including poor motivation.[77]

Most of these studies were conducted on populations where prolonged iodine deficiency occurs. The results, generally, were suggestive of neural impairment and poor sociopsychologic stimulation. These conclusions are consistent with the role that thyroid hormones have in ensuring proper mental development and functioning.

In light of the NHANES III study, the CDC recommended the monitoring of iodine intakes to determine whether this decrease was a "one-time" drop or a continuous fall in blood-iodine levels. The fact that the studies are nearly 20 years apart shows that there has been a continuous fall in iodine concentrations. The agency suggested that iodine excretion and dietary intake be routinely measured in health and dietary surveys, as part of an early warning system to prevent the reemergence of an iodine deficiency endemic—similar to the one that gripped the Midwestern United States at the turn of the 20th century.

During this period, many people who lived in the Midwest, in areas with iodine-deficient soils (areas far from the seashore) developed goiters. That region of the country became known as the "goiter belt." Iodized salt was introduced in 1922 to eradicate iodine deficiency. As the voluntary use of iodized salt rapidly spread, and as iodine was added to processed foods and milk products, the prevalence of goiter declined.[78]

Reductions in iodine intake became noticeable during the early 1980's when studies began to show drastic drops in UI levels. The decrease was thought to be due to the dairy industry's effort to reduce iodine in milk. Also, the replacement of iodine by bromine salts in dough conditioners throughout the commercial bread industry was considered another reason for the decrease in iodine use.[79] Researchers do not know whether the decrease in UI concentrations between NHANES I and III can be explained entirely by the changes in food production during the 1980's, or whether additional factors or trends that have not been measured are involved.

One such factor is the decrease in the use of iodized table salt. And, although the total consumption of iodized salt remains at about 50-60% of all salt consumed, the extent to which voluntary reduction in salt, used by segments of the population concerned about sodium intake and hypertension, has contributed to lower UI concentrations, is also unknown. Health researchers believe that should the intake of iodine continue to decrease, a portion of the population could become iodine deficient, resulting in the following consequences:

- *a reduction in the intellectual capacity of children born to mothers receiving insufficient amounts of iodine while pregnant; and*
- *a rise in the prevalence of iodine deficiency goiter and nodular goiter.*

The authors of the NHANES III-Iodine Study, did not make reference to the health implications caused by thyroid malfunctions. They resigned their concern to the dangers presented to children and fetuses. This was surprising, given the increased incidence of thyroid conditions, nationally.

Furthermore, the authors of NHANES III declared that they knew of no population-based studies, such as transient neonatal hypothyroidism, or recent goiter surveys that have shown health changes due to decreased iodine intake. This, however, does not prove that there is not a prevalence of either condition.

In response to this position, we can argue that such studies have not been warranted until now. The authors of this study and those assigned to monitor iodine-deficiency should consider two places where proof of iodine deficiency exists—the food industry and in medical reports that show an increased incidence of thyroid disease.

With respect to the food industry, the vast use of peanut- and soybean-based products throughout the food industry equates to an increased presence of goitrogens in the food chain. As noted, goitrogens inhibit iodine uptake and are, therefore, causes of iodine deficiency.

Health Alert: Increasing Incidence of Thyroid Disease

According to several medical reports, thyroid disease is now epidemic, affecting approximately 20 million Americans, and about 80% of them are women.[80] It was once thought that about eight million more people suffered from undetected thyroid problems.[81]

A recent study indicates that the number of people suffering from undetected thyroid problems is closer to 13 million. This study, the *Colorado Thyroid Disease Prevalence Study*,[82] set out to determine how common abnormal thyroid function actually is, and to look at the relationship between abnormal thyroid function, cholesterol levels, and thyroid symptoms.

The researchers studied 25,862 participants at the Colorado statewide health fair in 1995. Among those not taking thyroid medication, 8.9 percent were hypothyroid, while 1.1 percent were hyperthyroid. If taken as a sample population study, this would indicate that 9.9 percent of the population has unrecognized thyroid abnormalities. These figures suggest that, nationally, there might be 13 million Americans with an undiagnosed thyroid condition.

According to epidemiological studies, individuals at-risk for thyroid disease include infants that consume soy infant formula; women over 40; women who have recently given birth (within 6 months after delivery); people with high cholesterol; people experiencing depression; people who have had thyroid disease; people with a family history of autoimmune thyroid disease; and people who have been treated for hyperthyroidism. It is well known that hypothyroidism occurs five times more often in women than in men, with greater frequency in older individuals.[83]

Given the pervasiveness of peanuts and peanut by-products in the human food chain, these foods should be considered contributors to thyroid disease. Their role as iodine inhibitors must be urgently evaluated.

The next chapter describes the major chronic diseases associated with thyroid malfunction.

CHAPTER

9

Thyroid Malfunction Diseases

In Chapter 6, we reviewed the pathology of disease, specifically how any disruption of the body's two communication systems (nervous and endocrine) lead to illness and disease. When considering the fact that thyroid hormones affect nearly every cell and organ in the body, it is understandable that many major health ailments and diseases can be linked to a malfunctioning thyroid gland.

Although some research has linked thyroid disease to conditions, such as heart disease and depression, little has been published about the enormous role that thyroid disease plays in fostering other diseases. This chapter discusses the connection between thyroid gland malfunction and major illnesses and diseases, specifically, obesity, cancer, heart disease, diabetes, osteoporosis, menopause, and depression. And, because goitrogens are major contributors to thyroid malfunction and disease, nuts are major risk factors for these diseases. The notorious impact that nuts register against the human body—dismantling every molecular and biological process that support life—gives us an indication of how a meal of nuts can take five years away from the human life span. Five years equates to 60 months, 1,826 ¼ days, and 43,830 hours. This is a monumental loss of lifespan.

Thyroid-Obesity Connection

Obesity has reached epidemic proportion, gripping over 50% of the adult population and capturing dramatically larger numbers of children each year.[84] This condition is the leading risk factor for nearly every chronic disease, including coronary heart disease, stroke, diabetes mellitus, and certain cancers.[85]

The biological mechanisms that give rise to obesity are very controversial, and the methods used to treat it are even more controversial. Some researchers suggest that obesity develops as an interaction between a genetic predisposition and certain environmental factors, such as high-fat diets and low physical activity.

The notion of a genetic predisposition as a leading cause of obesity has led to the development and marketing of obesity drugs. A few of these drugs have caused greater harm than the good they were purported to produce. Unfortunately, such drugs continue to infiltrate the market.

The more acceptable causes of the obesity epidemic are the over consumption of food and lack of physical activity. Within this position, rest the most widely held belief that people are obese because they consume high intakes of fatty processed foods. However, most researchers overlook the contribution that natural foods make to obesity, specifically foods that contain toxins that impact metabolism. Goitrogens are foremost among these toxins.

Slowed Metabolism

The overall function of metabolism is to alter food into chemical components that aid in cell growth and energy utilization. There are two primary metabolic pathways. One pathway provides energy to tissues when needed. The other stores potential energy in times of energy excess. The pathway that generates energy is the catabolic (breakdown) pathway, while the pathway that stores energy is the synthetic or anabolic (build up) pathway. The anabolic pathway produces many of the compounds required for cells to grow and divide (i.e. proteins, lipids, and nucleic acids).

Researchers have confirmed that a slow metabolism is also a risk factor for obesity. When a person's metabolism is chronically slow, medical researchers refer to this condition as "habitual low energy-expenditure". *What exactly is this?*

Energy is expended in several ways. The most known is through physical exercise. Less known, is the burning of food energy through the thermic affect and basal metabolic rate. The thermic affect occurs when energy is burned while food is being ingested and digested. The basal metabolic rate or BMR is the rate of use of the body's energy. BMR is determined while the body is at rest, usually after an overnight fast or 14 hours after the last meal.

It has been proven that people who frequently exercise are not only able to burn excess energy, but when their bodies are at rest, their BMR is usually higher than those who do not exercise. As a result, they are usually able to fend off weight gain.

When the catabolic rate is slowed, much of the food energy is not immediately used to provide for the energy needs of the cell. The result is that this food energy is stored as fat, which leads to weight gain. This is why habitual low BMR has been a primary concern of health scientists researching the pathways of obesity. Within this research, the functionality of the thyroid gland is central to BMR.[86]

Researchers have learned that an inadequate production of thyroid hormones is often responsible for low habitual BMR because of the essential role that thyroid hormones play in cellular metabolism. This is also why excessive weight gain is a symptom of thyroid disease, specifically, hypothyroidism. In hypothyroidism, metabolism is slowed, causing nutrients to become excessive.

Excess nutrients are converted to fat. Again, it matters little whether or not the food is comprised of fat, because excess protein and starch are converted to fat and stored in the adipose tissue. According to health statistics, women are 5 to 8 times more likely than men to suffer from a thyroid condition.[80] This corresponds to the ever-increasing prevalence of obesity among women. The incidence of obesity among adult minority women has exceeded 50%, and obesity among Caucasian women is rising at a dramatic rate.

Pharmaceutical companies are attempting to respond to this crisis by producing drugs that target the thyroid; however, this effort is not only for profit's sake, but also exacerbates the problem. This subject is taken up in greater detail in Chapter 12.

The rise in obesity, particularly within the past decade, must be viewed along-side food industry changes. The food industry markets enormous amounts of goitrogen-infested peanut and soybean products and ingredients. Also, nutritionists have encouraged people to consume more nuts, and green vegetables that contain goitrogens. Women, in particular, have been the focus of nut promotion campaigns.

Generally, these dynamics have resulted in the consumption of goitrogens, increasing the occurrence of thyroid problems. The result has been epidemics of low BMR, leading to obesity. Obesity is, therefore, linked to the consumption of nuts, especially peanuts. And, considering that obesity is the principal risk factor of many chronic diseases, nuts must be viewed as major risk factors for chronic disease.

Thyroid-Cancer Connection

From the very outset, we must note two important facts with respect to cancer and its causes. First, the two major causes of cancer are smoking and improper dietary habits.[87] They combine for upwards of 70% of all cancer cases. This means that causes outside of our deliberate actions account for a small percentage of cancer incidences.

Those who tout genetic engineering as the solution to finding a cure for cancer are mistaken. Genetic engineering can only serve as an intervention, and this too, does not ensure that the person will avoid or be cured of cancer. As long as food is required for survival, cancer is an arm length away, because all cells, genetically-altered or otherwise, require nutrition for survival.

Secondly, cancer must also be understood in the context of how the two major causes of this disease bring it about. Smoking and food work at the molecular level. When a person inhales smoke—which does not contain protein, fats, and starches—the cell is being destroyed. Also, when a person consumes toxins, including plant poisons, the cell is being destroyed. In both instances, the ability of the cell to perform fails. This failure is seen as sudden cellular death or cellular dysfunction, leading to mutation. The latter leads to cancer.

Cancer, however, results from a continual alteration of critical regulatory genes that control cell proliferation, differentiation, and survival. So, unlike normal cells, cancer cells grow and divide in an uncontrolled manner, invading normal tissues and organs, and eventually spreading throughout the body. The generalized loss of growth control exhibited by cancer cells is often the result of accumulated abnormalities in multiple cell regulatory systems. Cancer, therefore, is not instantly acquired. It is a condition that gradually arises.

What are the regulatory systems that control cell activity? These regulatory systems are communication systems. All cells receive and respond to signals that dictate their behavior, and govern the activities that help them maintain their integrity; thus, sustaining the life of the organism. Communication is accomplished by a variety of signaling molecules. These molecules are secreted or expressed on the surface of cells, which then bind to receptors on the surface or in the nucleus of other cells. This process is termed "cell-to-cell signaling", and is divided into three general categories: endocrine signaling, paracrine signaling, and autocrine signaling.

Endocrine signaling occurs when the secreted hormone or neurotransmitter enters the bloodstream and is carried to a distant target cell. Paracrine signaling occurs when the secreted hormone or neurotransmitter acts on an adjacent cell in the same tissue. Autocrine signaling happens when the secreted hormone or neurotransmitter acts on the cell of origin.

In any of these signaling pathways, the binding of most signaling molecules to their receptors initiates a series of intracellular reactions that regulate virtually all aspects of cellular behavior, including metabolism, movement, proliferation, and differentiation. The molecular mechanisms responsible for the pathways of cell signaling has become a major area of research. In fact, interest in this area has been heightened by the fact that most cancers result from malfunctions in these signaling pathways. Also, many current insights into cell signaling mechanisms have come from the study of cancer cells.

Endocrine signaling is of great importance in cancer research. This form of signaling is facilitated by steroid and thyroid hormones. Steroid hormones include testosterone, estrogen, progesterone, and corticosteroids. Thyroid hormones include thyroxine and triiodothyronine.

Endocrine signaling hormones diffuse freely across the plasma membrane and enter the cell's nucleus. Once there, they bind to intracellular receptors. These receptors, which are members of a family of proteins known as the Steroid Receptor Superfamily, are transcription factors that contain domains for ligand binding, DNA binding, and transcriptional activation. *What is transcription?*

Transcription is the synthesis of a ribonucleic acid (RNA) molecule from a deoxyribonucleic acid (DNA) template. DNA contains the instructions that govern all cellular activities, and is carried in genes. These instructions or genes are managed through the synthesis of proteins from RNAs. Over-simplifying this relationship, the DNA code is transcribed or copied into a RNA molecule, then the RNA code is translated into amino acids, which builds the proteins used to carry out cellular activities.

Cellular behavior is not so much determined by the genes it inherits, in as much as it is dictated by the expression of those genes at any given time. The regulation of gene expression allows cells to adapt to changes in their environments and is responsible for the distinct activities of the multiple cell types.

The first step in the expression of a gene is the transcription of DNA into RNA. This is the primary level at which gene expression is regulated in cells. Once the RNA has been synthesized, it is modified in various ways to convert the primary transcript into its functional form. There are different types of RNA and each plays a distinct role in cell activity. Among these types are Messenger RNAs (mRNA), which serve as templates for protein synthesis; and Ribosomal RNAs (rRNA) and Transfer RNAs (tRNA), which play important roles in the function of mRNA translation. There are also other RNAs, which have important roles in splicing and protein sorting.

Transcription is controlled by proteins that bind to specific regulatory sequences. These proteins modulate the activity of RNA polymerase, the core component in transcription. Transcription factors, however, are dependent upon the binding action of endocrine signaling hormones. Therefore, endocrine hormones are principal components in the regulation of cellular activity.

For example, ligand binding determines whether transcription factors will serve as activators or repressors of target genes through their distinct effect on receptors. Some members of the steroid receptor superfamily, such as estrogen and glucocorticoid receptors, are unable to bind to DNA in the absence of the hormones. The binding of the hormones induce a conformational change in the receptor, allowing it to bind to regulatory DNA sequences and activate transcription of target genes.

Figure 11. DNA into RNA

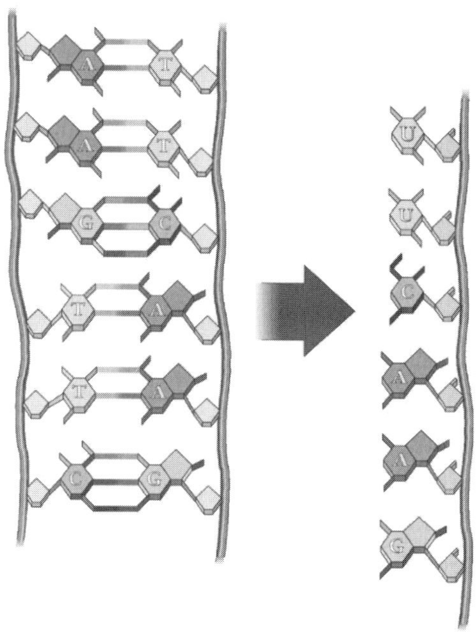

In other cases, the receptor binds DNA in either the presence or absence of the hormones, but hormone binding alters the activity of the receptor as a transcriptional regulatory molecule. For example, the thyroid hormone receptor (transcription factor) acts as a repressor in the absence of the hormone, but hormone binding converts it to an activator that stimulates transcription of thyroid hormone-inducible genes.

Given the vital role that hormones play in cellular health and survival, it is quite evident that any alteration in these processes leads to a malfunction in gene expression. Such a malfunction, at the greatest extent, leads to the development of cancer. *So, how do nut goitrogens produce cancer?*

Thyroid hormones are not only an intricate component in endocrine signaling, but are also primary components in the synthesis of cholesterol, which is used to construct steroid hormones. As noted, steroid hormones are also key signaling hormones that control transcription. Therefore, a dysfunctional thyroid gland, specifically one that produces low thyroid hormone output, is intrinsically involved in the development of cancer through its failure to synthesis thyroid and steroid hormones.

Figure 12. Thyroid Hormones in Transcription

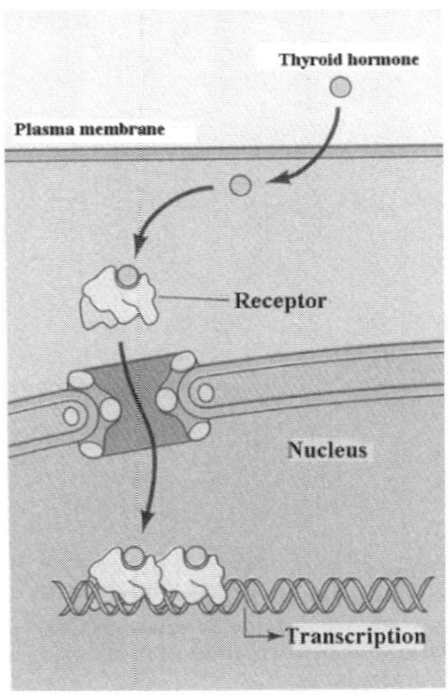

Goitrogens, however, deliver a one-two punch that makes them extremely high risk factors for cancer development. First, goitrogens rob the body of essential iodine. This, alone, inhibits the synthesis of thyroid hormones. Secondly, goitrogens cause thyroid hypertrophy, which threatens the overall continual function of the gland. Overall, nut goitrogens have the potential to cause long-termed and irreparable damage to the thyroid gland.

Thyroid-Heart Disease Connection

Ironically, nuts are highly touted as a food that reduces the risk of heart disease, yet the toxins contained in them are great promoters of heart disease. Nuts promote heart disease by impairing the thyroid gland's ability to produce the hormones that synthesizes cholesterol. According to biological pathways, the slightest thyroid abnormality can have a serious impact on long-term cardiac health.[88] Their contribution to heart disease is, therefore, noteworthy.

A survey conducted by the American Association of Clinical Endocrinologists (AACE), found that fewer than half of the adults who had been diagnosed with high cholesterol knew if they had ever been tested for thyroid disease, despite the well-documented connection between the two conditions. The survey revealed that nearly 90% of participants were unaware of the thyroid gland's impact on cholesterol regulation.

The thyroid-cholesterol connection has been well studied among health researchers. Studies have shown a direct correlation between the treatment of thyroid disease and the lowering of cholesterol levels.

As stated, poor dietary habits are leading causes of heart disease. People who consume foods high in fat are at significant risk, and the risk is magnified when such persons are also overweight and do not exercise. Thyroid disease ranks second to diet as a cause of high cholesterol. This is primarily due to the body's inability to metabolize cholesterol. This condition is known as hypercholesterolemia.

The metabolism of cholesterol is central to the thyroid gland, namely the thyroid hormones. Generally, thyroid hormones regulate body metabolism, so if the thyroid gland is underactive due to damage, or there is an inhibition of key substances such as iodine, the hormonal output is inadequate to maintain proper metabolism. Molecularly, it has been determined that thyroid hormones increases the rate of several important enzymes that control cholesterol metabolism.[89]

The average blood-cholesterol levels of persons with underactive thyroid glands are usually 250mg/dl or more, which is 30 to 50% higher than normal. Epidemiological studies suggests that ninety percent (90%) of people with diagnosed hypothyroidism have increased cholesterol or triglyceride levels, which in turn, increases their risk of heart disease.

An estimated 98 million Americans (more than half of American adults) have high cholesterol levels, making them candidates for heart disease. Heart disease, often referred to as coronary heart disease, accounts for more than 40% of all deaths in the United States, killing approximately 1 million people each year.[88] At least 50 million Americans have some form of cardiovascular disease, including high blood pressure. The American Heart Association estimates that an annual cost of nearly $300 billion stem from cardiovascular diseases.

Given these facts, nut goitrogens are principle risk factors for hypercholesterolemia and heart disease. *How many of the 98 million Americans estimated to have high blood-cholesterol eat nuts? How many will have their cholesterol levels driven up after following false dietary advice, stemming from bogus research that alleges health-promoting benefits of nuts?* Nut-promoting studies will only increase the incidence of heart disease.

Thyroid-Diabetes Connection

As noted in Chapter 6, diabetes is a disease characterized by an excessive amount of circulating glucose in the blood, which leads to an array of health implications. Currently, studies show that Type 2 diabetes develops from several pathways. Some studies have shown that diabetes is caused by inadequate production of insulin, which results from a malfunction or impaired pancreas. As such, little insulin is produced, so insulin injections are required. Other studies indicate that the body—for reasons not yet understood by scientists—resists the uptake of insulin. This condition is termed *insulin resistance.*

There is also the belief that diabetes often develops in obese persons because they have more adipose cells, which requires the pancreas' to output more insulin than it is capable of doing.[90] The logic is that the pancreas is biologically programmed to produce enough insulin to accommodate the needs of a preset number of cells, which is based upon the person's genetic code. An increase of cells, as is the case with obesity, places an extra burden on the pancreas—a burden that it has difficulty meeting.

Nut protease inhibitors and nut goitrogens, through their impairment of the pancreas and thyroid glands, respectively, produce the diabetic condition. In Chapter 7, we discussed the impact of protease inhibitors on the pancreas and how this impact causes the diabetic condition.

In the previous chapter, we learned that thyroid hormones are responsible for carbohydrate metabolism. The hormones stimulate glucose uptake and absorption in cells by working in concert with insulin. Therefore, a reduction in thyroid hormones caused by the goitrogenic inhibition of iodine, leads to a reduction in their interaction with insulin. This action causes diabetes.

This action is also the best explanation of the "insulin-resistance" theory in cells. However, the cells do not resist insulin in the elementary sense of the concept, but rather are incapable of using glucose because of low thyroid hormone output. Unfortunately, thyroid impairment is not atop medical researchers' list of factors that contribute to diabetes. The primary focus has been placed on the ingestion of starchy foods, while foods such as nuts are promoted as health foods, despite their biological assault on the thyroid and pancreas glands.

Thyroid-Osteoporosis Connection

Osteoporosis is characterized by low bone mass and structural deterioration of bone tissue, leading to bone fragility and an increased susceptibility to fractures. This disease refers to a group of diseases in which bone resorption outpaces bone deposit.

Bone is continuously broken down and replaced throughout life for the purposes of mobilizing calcium for systemic needs, and preventing the accumulation of old, fatigue-fractured material. This continuous cycle of bone formation and bone resorption is known as bone remodeling, a complex process regulated by many humoral and local factors. These factors have direct and indirect effects on bone structuring. The hormonal mechanisms of bone remodeling—deposit and resorption—reflects the interaction of parathyroid hormone (PTH), produced by the parathyroid glands, and Calcitonin, produced by the thyroid gland.

Parathyroid glands are located on the surface of the thyroid gland. There are four glands—two on each of the two thyroid gland lobes. They produce the parathyroid hormone (PTH). This hormone is released into circulation in response to a fall in blood calcium levels. Parathyroid hormone controls the concentration of calcium by acting on the kidneys and bones. In the kidneys, PTH stimulates the rate of resorption of calcium. Through its influence on the renal formation of active vitamin D metabolism, PTH influences the rate of absorption of calcium from the gastrointestinal tract. In bone, the hormone stimulates osteoclasts to resorb bone, which causes calcium release from bone matrix.

Figure 13. Parathyroid glands

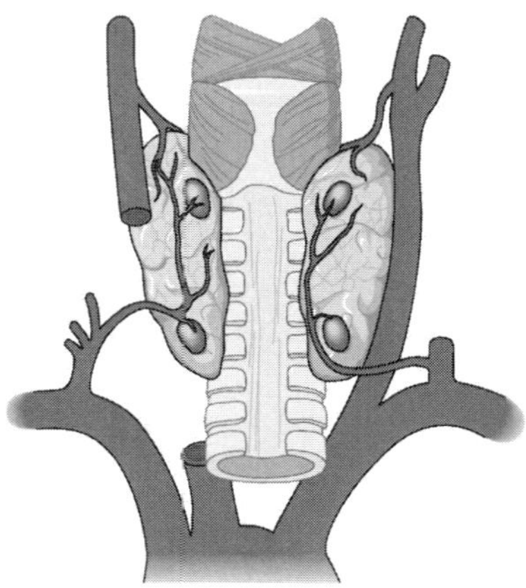

Calcitonin is a small polypeptide hormone produced by the parafollicular or "C" cells of the thyroid gland. It is secreted when blood calcium levels rise. It inhibits bone resorption and causes calcium to be deposited in the bones. It has also been hypothesized that calcitonin has a specific role after eating. Its secretion, induced by gastrointestinal peptide, results in greater skeletal retention of calcium, than would normally occur.

Because both parathyroid hormone and calcitonin are contained within the thyroid gland, any impairment to the gland, such as hypertrophy, compromises the production of these two hormones. For example, health researchers must consider these questions, *"Does thyroid disease significantly impact the production of calcitonin? Are the parathyroid glands impacted by thyroid cancer?*

The Role of Insulin and Sex Hormones

In addition to the calcium effects on bone produced by parathyroid hormone and calcitonin, insulin and sex steroids participate in many events that control bone formation and resorption. Insulin is a regulator of cartilage and bone growth, with both direct and indirect stimulative effects. It is known that untreated diabetic patients show bone and cartilage formation impairment, and often have a high incidence of osteoporosis.

Insulin also stimulates amino acid transport and RNA, collagen, and noncollagen protein synthesis in bone cultures. An indirect effect of insulin is derived from its regulation of the release of somatomedin (which stimulates DNA synthesis) by the liver. Insulin is also required for the normal mineralization of bone.

Clinical studies have long proven that a decrease in sex hormones—estrogen for women, and androgens for men—is associated with an increased incidence of osteoporosis. Cultured bone cells, as well as osteosarcoma cells, contain estrogen receptors that demonstrate metabolic changes when these receptors are activated.

And, although the precise action of estrogen's role in bone formation is yet under investigation, preliminary studies have shown that estrogen acts indirectly to alter the production of one or more of the local regulators of bone metabolism. This is validated through the use of hormone replacement therapy in menopausal women. This treatment, purportedly, decreases serum calcium, phosphate and urinary calcium levels, and produces retention of total body calcium.

The role of thyroid hormones in synthesizing sex hormones and the adverse action of nut goitrogens on thyroid hormone production have already been discussed.

Osteoporosis' Current Plight

Currently, osteoporosis is an important health problem in the United States, affecting approximately 24 million Americans—15 to 20 million of whom are women over 45 years of age. Millions of people already have the disease and millions of others have low bone mass, placing them at increased risk for osteoporosis.

Bone fractures are the major cause of morbidity and mortality associated with osteoporosis. The most common fractures are those of the forearm, hip, and vertebral body, as well as the humerus, tibia, pelvis, and ribs. Osteoporosis-related injuries result in complications leading to prolonged hospitalization, decreased independence, increased incidence of depression, and a reduced quality of life.

The disease takes an enormous personal and economic toll, with estimated costs in excess of $13.8 billion annually for direct medical treatment. The incidence of osteoporosis-related fractures is also increasing and constitutes a major public health problem in the United States.[91]

Research has suggested that after the fourth decade of life, bone reformation usually fails to completely replace the resorbed bone.[91] Therefore, bone turnover produces a net bone loss. Its rate, however, depends upon the frequency of remodeling cycles, and the imbalance between the amounts of bone resorbed and replaced at each remodeling cycle.

Therefore, women entering menopause and the elderly are at greater risk for the disease. According to studies, after the onset of menopause, bone loss in women increases substantially due to the reduced production of estrogen. Women can lose up to 20% of their total bone mass in 5 to 7 years following menopause.

Research also suggests that among the dietary factors that contribute to this disease, calcium plays an important role in preventing or delaying the onset of osteoporosis. It has been speculated that higher intakes of calcium could prevent 40 to 60 percent of osteoporosis-related bone fractures. Women are, therefore, encouraged to increase their intake of calcium. However, this has not been proven effective. As a result, drugs are being developed to treat the disease.

Several medications that treat postmenopausal women suffering from osteoporosis have been approved by the FDA. Drug combinations that feature chemically-concocted estrogen and parathyroid hormone are being carefully studied as possible treatment options.[92-93] Some have already entered the market.

In summation, several pathways that lead to osteoporosis have been confirmed. Calcitonin, PTH, thyroxine, and insulin are intrinsically involved in the regulation of calcium in bone reformation. It is evident that protease inhibitors' assault on the pancreas interferes with insulin production, making these poisons major contributors to osteoporosis. Additionally, goitrogens, which rob the thyroid of iodine, leads to a decreased production of both thyroid and steroid hormones, producing osteoporosis.

Additionally, the phytate content in nut's are known to rob the body of essential minerals, including calcium. This robbery also increases the risk of osteoporosis. The impact of nut phytates is covered in the next chapter.

Nuts are, therefore, major contributors to osteoporosis. And, considering that nut promotion is aimed at women, those predicting that this disease will rise dramatically in the next decade are, unfortunately, correct.

Thyroid-Menopause Connection

Mild hypothyroid symptoms are often mistaken for signs of menopause, aging or stress.[83] This, of course, does not mean that thyroid hormones do not have a role in either condition. In fact, thyroid hormones play a critical role in reproductive function. They work in concert with cholesterol to produce sex hormones. And, because female sex hormones are connected to menopause, thyroid hormones have a key role in menopause.

The sex hormones, testosterone (male) and estradiol (female), are secreted by the gonads and stimulate the development of secondary sex characteristics, and govern sexual function. The sex hormone-making process requires several mixed-function oxidations. The mitochondria of adrenal cells contain the enzyme desmolase, which catalyzes cholesterol, producing pregnenolone and isocaproic aldehyde. Pregnenolone is dehydrogenated to progesterone in the adrenal glands. Progesterone is the precursor of aldosterone, testosterone, and estradiol.

Menopause defines a point when menstruation ceases due to the loss of normal ovarian function. The ovaries contain structures called follicles that hold the egg cells. Women are usually born with approximately 2 million egg cells, but by puberty about 300,000 remain. Of these, only 400 to 500 mature to be released during the menstrual cycle. The rest degenerate over the years.

The menstrual cycle is regulated by the hypothalamus and pituitary. The pituitary gland generates hormones that causes the release of a new egg each month from its follicle. The follicle also increases production of the sex hormones estrogen, progesterone and adrogens, which thicken the lining of the uterus, preparing it to receive and nourish a fertilized egg following conception. When fertilization does not occur, estrogen and progesterone levels drop, the lining of the uterus breaks down, and menstruation occurs.

This cycle continues until the ovaries begin to decline due to falling hormone production, which usually begins when a woman reaches her mid-thirties. By her late forties, the decline accelerates, causing hormone levels to fluctuate. This causes irregular menstrual cycles. When a woman reaches her mid-fifties, her menstrual cycle usually ends.

According to the characteristics of menopause, the most dramatic physiological event is the decline in excretion rates of estrogen, leading to decreased circulating estrogen levels. Production rates for two of the major estrogens, estradiol, and estrone, decline. Circulating levels of estradiol drop from an average of 200pg/ml in young women with normal menstrual cycles to <30pg/ml in menopausal women.

The consequences of this decline is phenomenal. Estrogens and androgens affect many different tissues and organ systems throughout the body. For example, the brain, skeleton, bone marrow, heart and arteries, external genitalia, ovaries, breasts, muscle, skin, hair, liver, and kidneys are significantly impacted by estrogen. As a result, menopausal women experience symptoms that include sleep disturbances (due to hot flashes), sexual dysfunction (mainly a decrease in libido thought to be due to the decline in androgen levels), urogenial symptoms (e.g., vaginal dryness, irritation, and difficulty urinating), and psychological/somatic complaints such as depression, mood swings, irritability, and an overall diminished sense of well being.

Epidemiological data also suggest that the risk for several serious health disorders increase after a woman enters menopause.[94] Such disorders include osteoporosis, cardiovascular disease, Alzheimer's disease, macular degenerative diseases, thyroid disease, and breast and colon cancer. These risks stem from changes in the hormonal environment that occur with menopause.

Other studies suggest that risk for chronic diseases, such as Alzheimer's disease, macular degeneration, and colon cancer may be related to hypoestrogenism. Given this, it has been assumed that estrogen replacement may decrease the risk for these diseases. Hormone replacement therapy (HRT) is the primary modality in the treatment of menopause-related symptoms.

HRT entails the use of pharmaceuticals—estrogens, progestins, and androgens—as a treatment for the short term complaints related to hormone deficiency, and as preventive therapy for serious health problems such as osteoporosis and CVD. There are, however, numerous side effects associated with the use of HRT, many of which are linked to the long-term use of this treatment.

Women who use HRT often experience bloating, breast tenderness, weight gain, headaches, nausea, irritability, and premenstrual-like symptoms. Women also experience uterine bleeding, and are at an increased risk of uterine cancer.[95] Those who have had a continuous daily estrogen/progestin regimen over six months are much more likely to experience amenorrhea.

There are other well-documented complications from the use of HRT. These include an increase in the risks of breast cancer;[96] incidence of venous thromboembolism; [97] an increase in serum triglyceride levels; and an increase in gallbladder disease.[95]

Despite drug therapies, health scientists admit that it is yet unclear why estrogen production in the ovaries begin to decline when women enter their thirties. Little research has been focused on the potential impact of dietary regimens as a cause for menopause. However, if diet is central to health conditions that result from menopause, such as heart disease, then diet also should have a major stake in causing menopause. *So, how do nuts increase the risk of menopause?*

Thyroid hormones significantly impact the production of sex hormones. This impact is either through the thyroid hormone's role in metabolism or in the synthesis of cholesterol, a precursor for sex hormones. Obviously, low thyroid hormone availability is responsible for decreases in estrogens and other cholesterol-based hormones. This makes nut goitrogens a leading risk factor for menopause.

Thyroid-Depression Connection

According to leading endocrinologists, thyroid disease is often misdiagnosed as depression.[98] Both conditions have overlapping symptoms, which include apathy, sadness, and fatigue. A nationwide study revealed that despite these commonalities, only one in five Americans with symptoms of depression is tested for thyroid disease.[80] The presumption is that millions of people with depressive symptoms may actually suffer from thyroid disease.

Depressive illnesses are among the most prevalent psychiatric disorders in adults. The distinction between depressive illness and the emotional downward mood swings that everyone experiences as part of daily living, lies in the severity and persistency of symptoms. The former occurs every day for, at least, 2 weeks in duration and is accompanied by noticeable changes in social and occupational functioning.

Figure 14. Synapse

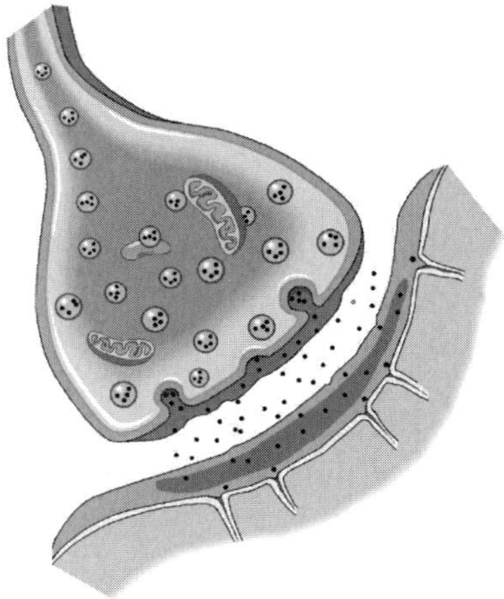

Depressive disorders are defined as unipolar and bipolar. People with unipolar depression only experience depressed moods. Those suffering from bipolar depression experience manic-depressive disorders, which are characterized by periods of euphoric moods and dementia. Unipolar depression is the most common form of depression. There are several at-risk populations for unipolar depression. Among these populations are women between the ages of 35 and 45 years.

Estimates of point of prevalence (the proportion of the population with the diagnosis at a point in time) for unipolar depression are 2-3% in adult males and 5-9% in adult females, with a lifetime risk of 8-12% for men and 20-26% for women.

Clinical depression is determined by multiple factors, including biological, psychological and interpersonal factors. Biologically, research in brain neurochemistry has led to two prominent hypotheses about the underpinnings of depressive disorders.

The first is the biogenic-amine theory, which holds that mood is regulated in the brain by complex chemicals functioning as transmitters in the synapse between cells. In brain function, messages between brain cells occur via the release of neurotransmitters across the synapse. The messages are then completed by means of a two-stage process in which the biogenic amines are taken back into the transmitting cell and rendered inactive by specific enzymes. It is believed that major depressive disorders, and possibly other forms of depression, result from deficiencies in the availability of certain neurotransmitters to the postsynaptic nerve cell.

Another hypothesis views depression as the result of abnormalities in cells that interfere with the cells' ability to receive messages from neurotransmitters. These postsynaptic cells, it is speculated, have developed an overabundance of specific receptors, which causes a chronic underproduction of biogenic amines and leaves the person vulnerable to depressed moods. The neurotransmitters norepinephrine, serotonin, and acetylcholine are among the amines conceptualized to be central to depression.

Despite these two theories, research has demonstrated the role that thyroid hormones play in brain neurotransmission. Thyroid hormones concentrate neurotransmitters and receptors, and as such, significantly influences neurotransmission. Given this, a decrease in thyroid hormone production, such as that which results from the ingestion of peanut goitrogens, adversely affects neurotransmission. This makes the consumption of nuts a risk factor for depressive illnesses.

Recent research, however, has verified a more intricate relationship between the brain and thyroid hormones. Biological studies have confirmed that thyroid hormones act as neurotransmitters or as molecules that help transmit information within the brain.[99] In Chapter 6, we discussed the dual role of hormones and neurotransmitters—as hormones can act as neurotransmitters and vice versa.

During brain development in the fetus, and before the neurotransmission function has been established, many neurotransmitters act as growth regulators and hormones. When these neurotransmitters mature in their roles and adapt to memory requirements, growth-related processes remain their responsibility. Catecholamines, such as noradrenaline (the brain's version of adrenaline), demonstrate this type of behavior, and research indicates that thyroid hormones also cross over in the adult brain and behave like neurotransmitters.

The thyroid hormone, thyroxine, has been shown to be concentrated in the brain's noradrenergic centers (where there is noradrenaline), including the locus coeruleus (a control center of the brain located at the base of the neck behind the cerebellum). New structural data has permitted researchers to understand the thyroid hormone circuitry in the locus coeruleus. High concentrations of noradrenaline in the locus coeruleus are now known to actively help convert thyroid hormones, making the locus coeruleus a preeminent site for thyroxine concentration.

This research establishes thyroid hormones as neurotransmitters, and that the noradrenaline and thyroid hormone circuitry are interconnected. Thus, there exists a direct connection between these systems, supporting the idea that thyroid hormones serve as co-transmitters with noradrenaline in the nervous system. Figuratively, this means that noradrenaline and thyroid share information and co-transmit. This, again, reinforces the fact that thyroid hormones are vital to all biological and neurological functions.

Given the vital importance of thyroid hormones to proper brain function, nut goitrogens are risk factors for depressive disorders. Perhaps this is why this vegetation is called *nuts*.

CHAPTER

10

Danger of Nut Phytates

In the previous chapters, we addressed the adverse biological impact caused by the poisonous protease inhibitors and goitrogens contained in nuts. Now we turn our attention to the mineral-binding poisons contained in nuts. The mineral-binding or phytate content binds to minerals such as iron, calcium, magnesium and zinc. The phytate content is also heat-stable and, therefore, remains intact despite cooking or normal heat treatment methods. This chapter addresses the adverse health impact registered by this class of poisons.

As stated, trace elements or minerals are essential to the body's homeostatic regulation. And, because the amount of trace elements found in the body is relatively minute, anything that interferes with their uptake threatens the life of the organism. Among the many minerals required by the body, iron, magnesium, calcium and zinc have been among the most studied, and several diseases have been linked to their deficiencies. This chapter describes the function of these minerals and the adverse health impact caused by their deficiencies.

Impact of Iron Deficiency

Iron forms the core constituent of the red blood cells, specifically hemoglobin. Iron is contained in all heme and nonheme cellular compartments. Haem proteins include hemoglobin, myoglobin, and cytochromes. Hemoglobin transports oxygen to body tissues, while myoglobin ensures that there is an adequate oxygen supply during muscle contraction.

Cytochromes are a group of haem-containing electron transport enzymes that are essential for the generation of adenosine triphosphate (ATP). As previously noted, ATP is the most important chemical form of energy in cells and is used to drive metabolic processes.

In mitochondria, nonheme compounds account for more iron than do those containing heme. Nonheme compounds are also used for an array of enzymatic functions. Therefore, iron deficiency leads to a reduction in the iron content of all heme and nonheme compartments. The physiological consequences of iron deficiency are related to both impaired oxygen delivery and reduced metabolic tissue iron.

Anemia, the most common condition associated with iron deficiency, is caused by reduced hemoglobin synthesis, which results in a reduced availability of oxygen to all body cells. A consequence of anemia is the accumulation of carbon dioxide in cells, which causes decreased efficiency of both cellular and organ functions.

Tissue iron deficiency leads to mucosal and epithelial abnormalities; impaired immunity, leading to infections; skeletal muscle dysfunctions; and behavioral and neurological abnormalities. Symptoms of iron deficiency include pale skin, abnormal fatigue, shortness of breath, depression, low blood pressure, sciatic rheumatism, dizziness, and a loss of interest in sex.

The iron inhibitory affects of nuts due to their phytate content has been well documented.[47] All nuts, including peanuts, walnuts, almonds, and hazelnuts, were found to contain significant amounts of two known inhibitors of iron absorption.

Iron deficiency is common in developing countries where staple diets largely consist of legumes and cereals, which have high phytate contents.[100] Unfortunately, iron deficiency has risen in the United States. According to a study published by the American Medical Association, one out of ten women and small children are iron deficient. Researchers at the National Center for Health Statistics (NCHC) have estimated that 700,000 toddlers and 7.8 million women are iron deficient, and of those, approximately 240,000 toddlers and 3.3 million women have anemia.

There are many causes for the prevalence of iron deficiency in the United States—one of which is the proliferation of nuts and soy-based products (both containing high phytate contents) in the market. And, nut promoting studies are certain to increase iron deficiency.

Impact of Calcium Deficiency

Calcium is the body's most abundant mineral. Ninety-nine percent of the calcium in the body is deposited in bones and teeth with the remainder found in the soft tissues. Calcium is essential for proper bone development and normal blood clotting. It also helps maintain a balance between sodium, potassium and magnesium, and is essential for the proper utilization of phosphorus and vitamins A, C and D.

As previously discussed, calcium deficiency leads to osteoporosis. Other ailments associated with calcium deficiency include muscle cramps, numbness and tingling in arms and legs, brittle nails, joint pains, tooth decay, nervousness, mental depression, irritability, and Parkinson's disease.

The ever-increasing epidemic of osteoporosis among women has raised concerns about calcium deficiency. Health researchers have failed to identify dietary factors that contribute to calcium deficiency. The focus has been placed on the need for calcium supplements or increased calcium intake, but not on the factors that rob the body of calcium. The consumption of foods containing phytates is among those factors.

The consumption of nut protease inhibitors and goitrogens increases the risk for osteoporosis. When nut phytates are added to the equation, this makes the consumption of nuts a major risk factor for calcium deficiency and osteoporosis.

Meanwhile, medical institutions are following broadly held assumptions that nuts are nutritious foods and, as a result, are encouraging women to consume them. This, again, sheds light on the harmful impact of false nutritional advice.

Impact of Zinc Deficiency

Zinc is an important trace element in human nutrition. It is an essential mineral found in most tissues of the body. The kidney, liver, pancreas, and spermatozoa have the highest concentrations of zinc. This mineral has several important roles:

- *Zinc influences the entire hormonal system and all the glands, especially the prostate gland.*
- *Zinc is essential for the formation of RNA and DNA, and also for the synthesis of body protein.*
- *Zinc affects tissue respiration by its participation in carbonic amyldrase, which transports carbon dioxide from the tissues to the blood.*
- *Zinc is essential for growth and normal functioning of the sex organs and and the Prostate gland.*
- *Zinc increases the rate of burn and wound healing.*
- *Zinc normalizes insulin in the blood and, in so doing, is recommended in some types of diabetes treatments.*
- *Zinc has a role in reducing blood-cholesterol levels.*

Metabolically, zinc participates in ligand binding with organic molecules; and is therefore, ubiquitous in sub-cellular metabolism. For example, zinc is essential for gene expression and nucleic acid metabolism, which accounts for its importance in cellular growth and differentiation. Its ligand binding properties are utilized effectively at the catalytic site of a wide range of enzymes. Zinc also has many structural roles in biological membranes, cell receptors, enzymes and other proteins.

Given zinc's critical role, a lack of it causes a disruption of biological systems that are linked to several major diseases. As a component in cellular binding and transcription activities, a lack of zinc can lead to cellular malfunction. Zinc deficiency can also cause retarded growth, birth defects, hypogonadism, impaired sexual function, loss of fertility, enlargement of the prostate gland, lowered resistance to infection, slow healing of wounds, and skin diseases. A zinc deficiency can cause hair loss, dandruff, apathy and a loss of interest in learning.

Impact of Magnesium Deficiency

Approximately half of the magnesium in the body is located in the bones. There, it combines with calcium and phosphorus to ensure the strength and firmness of the bones and teeth. Magnesium is also located in the muscles, red blood cells, and other soft tissue.

Magnesium is an important catalyst in many enzyme reactions, especially those involved in energy production. Magnesium also helps in the utilization of vitamins B and E, calcium, fats, and other minerals. It is effective in reducing cholesterol levels and in this respect, is considered helpful in preventing heart attacks.

When magnesium is deficient, kidney and gall bladder stones can occur. Irritability, confusion, depression, impaired protein metabolism, and premature wrinkles also occur. A lack of this mineral can also cause over-calcification of the joints, leading to rheumatoid arthritis.

A Priority Consideration

Based upon the importance of trace elements to the human body, the pervasiveness of phytates in the human food chain via nuts and soybeans must be carefully evaluated. This becomes more important because both nuts and soybeans are highly touted as nutritious foods, and are firmly recommended by nutritionists.

CHAPTER 11

Nut Allergen Hazards

Food allergies have risen among the American population. Both adults and children are under the burden of this increasing epidemic. Most of the allergies are due to proteins found in milk, eggs, and nuts, especially peanuts. Studies have shown that about 25% of Americans believe they have food allergies that cause a broad range of minor conditions including fatigue, depression, and irritability.[101]

What is a food allergy? A food allergy occurs when whole food proteins or other large molecules cross the intestinal lining and enter the body tissues. This elicits a biological reaction, especially since proteins are usually degraded into amino acids before passing through the intestinal lining. After penetrating the intestines and entering the blood stream, the body responds to allergens, viewing them as dangerous intruders. The body mobilizes its forces—antibodies and histamines-—to fend off the allergens.

Allergic reactions are biochemical and biological events that can result in mild or severe health conditions, and for this reason, they are viewed as serious threats to human health. An allergic reaction comprises two components in the immune system. One is the production of immunoglobulin E (IgE), a type of antibody that circulates throughout the blood. The other is the mast cell, a specific cell that occurs in all body tissues but is especially common in areas of the body that are typical sites of allergic reactions, such as the nose, throat, lungs, skin, and gastrointestinal tract.

Allergy Pathway

Before an allergic reaction can occur, a person must first be exposed to the food allergen. When this food allergen passes the intestinal lining, it triggers certain cells to produce specific IgE antibodies in large amounts. IgE antibodies are made by the B cells, with assistance from T cells, on the first encounter with an antigen. The antigen-specific IgE molecules bind to mast cells, which are granular connective tissue cells that contain histamine and other chemical mediators. The mast cells are present in large numbers in the mucous membranes, the skin, nose, mouth, eye, respiratory tract and gut.

On the body's next encounter with the antigen, the antigen interacts with the specific IgE antibodies and there is an explosive degranulation of the mast cells. Histamine and other mediators such as serotonin and leukotrienes are released. These substances act on blood vessels, mucous glands and smooth muscle, causing the symptoms of the allergy.

Depending upon the tissue in which these chemicals are released, the person will experience various symptoms of food allergy. For example, if the mast cells release chemicals in the ears, nose, and throat, a person may feel an itching in the mouth, and may have trouble breathing or swallowing. If the affected mast cells are located in the gastrointestinal tract, the person may have abdominal pain or diarrhea. These chemicals, when released by skin mast cells, can cause hives.

Allergic reactions can range from mild symptoms to serious health conditions, including shock. Anaphylaxis is an acute systemic allergic reaction that involves the entire body. It is the most serious form of allergic reaction because normal body functions are disrupted to the extent that the person can die. An anaphylaxis reaction is sudden and severe.

In an anaphylaxis occurrence, the immune system releases histamines and antibodies, which cause muscle contractions and constriction of the airways. The person experiences wheezing and difficulty breathing. Gastrointestinal symptoms such as abdominal pain, cramps, vomiting, and diarrhea also occur.

The histamine that is released causes the blood vessels to dilate, which lowers blood pressure. Fluid also leaks from the bloodstream into the tissues, which lowers the blood volume. This causes shock. Shock is the major cause of death from anaphylaxis, although swelling of the vocal cords can also cause death.

Figure 15. Allergy Pathway

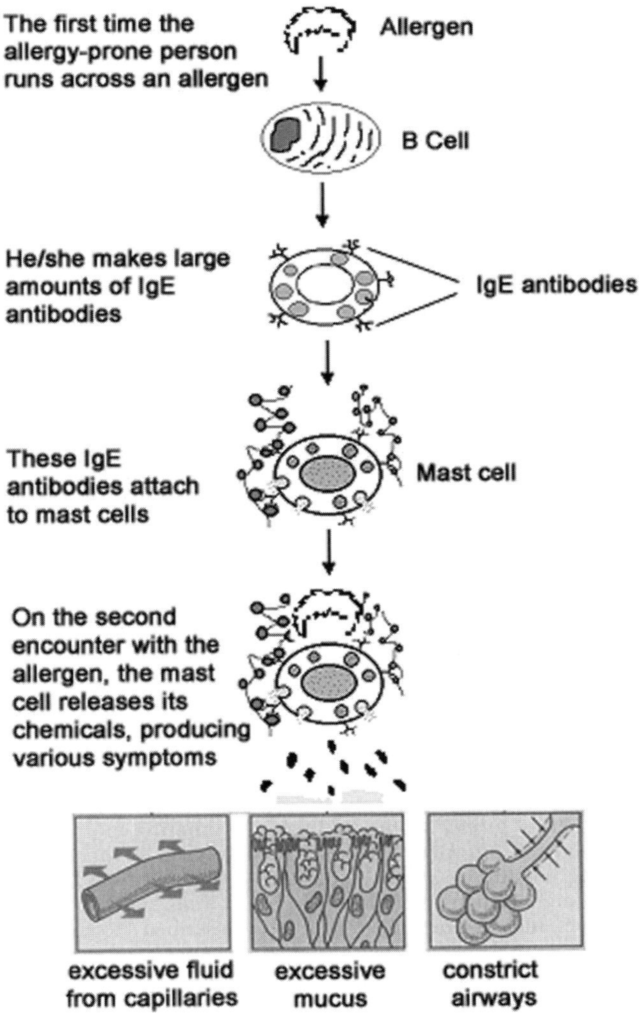

Fluid can also leak into the alveoli (air sacs) of the lungs causing pulmonary edema. Hives and angioedema (hives on the lips, eyelids and throat) also occur. Angioedema may be severe enough to cause obstruction of the airway.

Nut Allergens

The protein content of nuts have long been known to contain allergens, and those frequently implicated include almonds,[102] Brazil nuts,[103] cashews,[104] hazelnuts,[105] macadamia nuts[104], pecans, pine nuts[106], pistachios, and walnuts.[107] Most of these allergens are heat-stable and are characterized by their ability to cause severe allergic reactions. Nearly all nuts have elicited either fatal or near-fatal allergic reactions. For example, almonds[108], Brazil nuts,[109] cashews,[110] pistachios,[111] and pecans,[112] are responsible for allergic reactions that have resulted in fatalities. Ingestion of hazelnuts,[107] pine nuts,[113] pistachios,[114] and walnuts,[107] have resulted in cases of near-fatal reactions.

The allergencity of peanuts have been known since 1920. To date, the peanut is one of the most prevalent food allergens in North America.[101] Peanut allergy is a major health problem in the United States because they are ubiquitous in the contemporary diet of children and teenagers. Furthermore, they are used as a cheap source of protein in many processed foods. This situation has lead to early sensitization, often resulting in life-long sensitivity.

Peanuts are also responsible for the most common causes of severe allergic reactions in the United States. In several reviews of fatal or near-fatal anaphylaxis to foods, peanuts were implicated in the majority of the cases. In one study, 13 food-induced anaphylactic reactions—6 fatal and 7 near-fatal—in children were recorded from three cities over a 14 month period.[107] Peanuts were the most frequently implicated food in the fatal cases. Tree nuts were most common in the near-fatal reactions.

As a result of the "peanut problem", some institutions have issued food alerts with respect to peanut allergens.[115] Pediatric organizations are very concerned with the ever-increasing prevalence of peanut-induced allergies among children.[116] Pregnant and breastfeeding women have been warned not to eat peanuts.[117] This advice is being issued to women who either suffer themselves or whose families suffer from health conditions including asthma, eczema, hay fever or other allergies.

Some organizations have considered banning peanuts, altogether.[118] Several school districts have engaged preventive measures—one of which is to separate students that are allergic to peanuts and monitor their lunch and snack periods to ensure that they are not ingesting peanuts or foods with peanuts in them.[119] This is generally deemed the most effective approach, especially considering the fact that not all peanut allergens have been identified.

According to the American Peanut Council, the peanut is a complex plant food, having more than 30 different proteins that can serve as allergens. Recent research, however, has identified several peanut protein allergens.[120] Two of these proteins, *Ara h I* (MW 63.5kD) and *Ara h II* (MW 17 kD), have been isolated and characterized as major peanut proteins. Serum from more than 90% of peanut-allergic patients have been found to contain specific IgE to these two fractions. These allergens are heat stable, as in-vitro chemical denaturation (mimicking digestion) was found to only partially denature the proteins. This is the nature of food allergens. Again, food proteins are normally degraded by the heat of cooking, or by stomach acids and enzymes that digest food.

As an effort to address the peanut allergy problem, medical researchers are working on developing treatments to prevent or decrease symptoms. Immunotherapy treatments to desensitize individuals are also being explored. Oral vaccinations are being developed by leading universities such as John Hopkins University of Medicine. This effort is consistent with the downward trends of modern medicine, which is to concoct chemical drugs to combat the adverse reactions caused by the chemicals in foods—particularly foods that should not be in the human food chain.

According to research, tree nut hypersensitivity is most prominent in adults because of the later introduction of nuts into the human diet and the life-long sensitivity to these antigens.[121] The American Peanut Council agrees that peanut allergy is progressive and that subsequent reactions tend to be more severe. Nonetheless, the promotion of peanuts as a nutritious and healthy food continues. This also calls attention to the nut-promoting research that is targeted toward the adult population. Given this, there is a foreseeable rise in adult allergies as a result of the increased consumption of nuts.

CHAPTER 12

Pharmaceutical Seizure

The promotion of nut consumption through "advertisement" studies has been a force driving the chronic disease epidemic. The previous chapters described the numerous diseases that result from nut consumption. The enormous impact that nuts register is further validated through the monumental financial success of the pharmaceutical industry.

According to Promotional Insights,[122] a periodical that tracts marketing and advertising spending, pharmaceutical companies spent record amounts on advertisements in 1999. Promotional expenditures climbed nearly 12%, to $7.8 billion. Detail spending increased 7%, to $5.8 billion; event spending grew nearly 30%, to $1.7 billion.

As a result of this monumental financial output—for the purpose of cashing in on the ill-health of the population—physicians in the United States wrote an average of 2,060 prescriptions each in 1999.[123] This was up by 9 percent from 1998. Primary care physicians wrote more than half (53.5 percent) of all prescriptions dispensed by U.S. retail pharmacies.

Leading the way as the most prescribed medication was The Knoll's hyperthyroidism nostrum, Synthroid. Pfizer/Warner-Lambert's Lipitor, which is used to reduce blood-lipid levels, was second, followed by Wyeth-Ayerst's Premarin tablets, an estrogen replacement narcotic. The ranking of these drugs is evidence of the rise of molecular and biological malfunctions that, among other factors, stem from a distressed thyroid gland.

Each of these drugs were concocted to directly or indirectly treat the health ailments that are linked to the thyroid gland and thyroid hormones. In Chapter 8, we learned that thyroid hormones have the major role in cholesterol metabolism, which among several vital processes, control blood-lipid levels and sex hormone production. Therefore, any disruption in cholesterol metabolism leads to high LDL levels and low sex hormone production.

The majority of those taking these toxic nostrums are women. When considering that women are also being advised to eat the very thing (nuts) that reduces thyroid hormone production, it is evident that women are being grossly misguided. This destructive situation is further exacerbated when the drugs produce complications that threaten the lives of those taking them. Meanwhile, profits are soaring for both the nut and drug industries. The following sections describe the health hazards rendered by each drug.

Synthroid

Synthroid is a synthetic thyroid hormone that the drug maker claims is identical to the hormone produced by the thyroid gland. Yet, the drug is made in a laboratory and not in the thyroid gland. *How is it identical?* The drug can be prescribed in eleven different strengths or dosages. Clearly, its administration is radically different from the administration of hormones by the thyroid gland. A patient's doctor is charged with prescribing the "right" dosage. This makes trial-and-error a constant occurrence.

There are numerous health threats associated with Synthroid. These include nervousness, irritability; headache; insomnia; diarrhea, and menstrual irregularities. Figure 10 describes more severe side effects experienced by a woman. She gives a thorough description of how the side effects have impacted her health.[124]

Figure 16. Pleading Synthroid User

"I have been on Synthroid now for the past 4+ years. I have noted the following some of which have become progressively worse:

First, I have been on (.75mcg) of Synthroid and 3 weeks ago was bumped up to (.88mcg). Since this increase I have more energy, but I am experiencing "profuse" hair loss!!! I had some hair loss before this increase, but nothing like this! Is there an adjustment period for the dosage increase, or is this dosage too strong? Does this ever stop? Anyone else experience an increase in hair loss when Synthroid dosage was increased?

Below are other problems noted from the last 4 years. Some of these occurred before the Synthroid and have continued or have become worse; others are new problems since being on the Synthroid:

Weight gain, hair loss, fibromylgia and other unexplained muscle and joint aches, feeling cold or feeling hot, low grade fevers, skin itching, small tiny itching bumps on abdomen/legs/arms that resemble tiny bug bites, dry skin, dry hair, thinning lashes and brows, swollen eyes, insomnia, swollen glands in the neck, extremely heavy periods, thickened cervical mucus, an very small area on the side of my head that feels like a bump (but there is nothing there) that has a intermitted tingling pressure and hurts when pressed on and especially at the time when I ovulate and/or start my period or get stressed, don't handle stress as well, hand tremors, color changes in facial skin - reddening of the face, easy bruising, rapid growing fingernails, lethargic, forgetfulness, difficulty concentrating, calcifications on hip joints, salivary duct stones, irregular pulse, extreme fatigue, tingling in hands/fingers/feet, need I go on..."

Much of what the woman experienced is common with thyroid conditions, yet she is taking a drug that is, supposedly, a remedy for thyroid problems. One would think that after four years of using Synthroid, her health would have improved, but this is not the nature of drugs.

Drugs, such as these, are prescribed for many years, even lifetimes. Through it all, the body is never healed. Additionally, the body develops a dependency on the drug as it attempts to adjust. When people choose to stop using the drug, they experience withdrawal symptoms that are usually much worst and longer in duration than the illness might have been had they chose a safer method, such as modifying their lifestyle habits.

Lipitor

Lipitor lowers cholesterol by inhibiting the enzyme in the liver responsible for cholesterol metabolism. The manufacturer claims that Lipitor is able to reduce circulating LDL levels by up to 60%, and triglyceride levels by up to 40%. Lipitor currently is the most potent drug per milligrams in the class of cholesterol-lowering nostrums.

Although the drug maker declares Lipitor to be "generally well tolerated", it is known to cause constipation, diarrhea, ingestion, gas, nausea, headache, and muscle aches. Some patients will experience marked muscle inflammation, which necessitates stopping the drug. This drug also significantly affects the liver and kidney, so people with conditions related to these organs are advised to use Lipitor with extreme caution.

The manufacturer does not define "well tolerated". Perhaps "well tolerated" means that the person will not need emergency care or suffer sudden death. *How can these side effects be considered tolerable?* The body certainly does not tolerate them, and this is demonstrated in its response. These side effects are serious conditions because they disrupt overall digestion. *Furthermore, does not a drastic reduction in blood-lipid levels also compromise sex hormone production?* It appears that women taking Lipitor are on their way to taking Premarin.

Premarin

Premarin is a conjugated estrogen that is prescribed to prevent and manage osteoporosis, severe vasomotor symptoms, and vaginal dryness—ailments associated with menopause. As with the other leading drugs, the risk factors associated with this chemical concoction are enormous. Side effects that can occur through the use of this nostrum include cancer of the uterus, blood clots, nausea, vomiting, breast tenderness, interference with blood-sugar levels, headache, breakthrough bleeding, spotting, weight changes, and swelling of fingers and ankles.

Premarin was touted as a drug that prevents heart disease and osteoporosis. However, there is now evidence that Premarin does not prevent heart attacks and can actually raise triglycerides. It does not prevent osteoporosis. At best, it may slow bone loss by 2.5%. On the other hand, a January 2000 study by the National Cancer Institute found that women increase their risk of breast cancer by 10% for each year they take Premarin.

A Priority Consideration

While those taking the drugs experience the awesome ailments associated with them, drug manufacturers continue to rake in enormous profits. For example, Lipitor is the market leader in a "cholesterol and triglyceride reducer" market that increased by more than 23% in 1999, amounting to $10.44 billion. Lipitor accounted for 27% of the total market with sales of almost $3 billion. This is up from the 20.8% of the market it had in 1998, which generated $1.76 billion in sales.

When considering the vital role of cholesterol, researchers and drug makers are apparently ignoring two popular pathways that lead to high blood-lipid levels. One, of course, is improper cholesterol metabolism. The other is the over consumption of foods, especially fatty foods. Each of these conditions can be remedied by correct modifications to diet. *So, what purpose does Lipitor really serve? What purpose do any of these drugs serve when the root of the problem is diet?*

The sad truth is that no one is ever healed by drugs. People will, once again, find themselves revisiting diet and exercise as the best solutions, especially after the brutal failure experienced as a result of taking drugs. And, because this cycle has been the trend, efforts must be made to properly educate all—health practitioners, nutritionists, and the general public—about the correct diet for humans. High on the list is education about foods, specifically the identification of foods that are fit for humans from those that are unfit.

CHAPTER

13

Food Distinctions Required

This book, to a notable extent, has proven that nuts are unfit for human consumption. The naturally-occurring toxins contained in nuts are hazardous to humans when ingested. However, because this hazard is not an "instant combustion" into sickness, many are prone to dismiss it as noncritical. Therefore, some people might continue to consume them, arguing that their parents ate nuts and yet lived 60 or 70 years.

Such a position frustrates any attempt to recommend better eating habits. Furthermore, the fact that a person lived 65 or 70 years does not substantiate their diet as suitable for human nutrition. *How many more years could that person have enjoyed if nuts were eliminated from his or her diet?* And, if that person lived 70 years, how many of those years were spent in agony because of health ailments. These questions are rarely considered when the lifespans of others are boasted.

This position also does not consider the disease-nutrition connection. Many fail to blame their dietary habits when they are afflicted with disease, yet it is disease that has made the average lifespan a mere 70 or so years. We should not be deceived into believing that such a lifespan is long.

If today's disease burden could be alleviated, might not the average lifespan be 170 years instead of 70 years? If this seems ridiculous, how might those who lived in the early 1900's—when the average lifespan was between 40 and 50 years—view the climb to 70 years? They would probably appreciate the progress.

When considering the potential lifespan of humans, the foremost question is: *"How meticulous does one's diet have to be to live a disease-free life?"* A disease-free life would equate to a lifespan that would boggle the mind—150, 200, or 300 years. Again, some might consider this farfetched, but the scientists who are on the fringes of longevity research agree that humans have the capacity to live, at least, twice as long as today's average lifespan.[125] The Honorable Elijah Muhammad declares that humans have the potential to live nearly 1,000 years. This, of course, is a vast subject, but suffice it to state that any attempt to live a long and disease-free life must include the elimination of toxic foods from one's diet.

On several instances throughout this book, we discussed the need to confirm food distinctions. This, realistically, is at the core of good health and longevity. In our pursuit of this objective, we must first ask, *"Who or what determines the vegetation that we refer to as vegetables—the vegetation earmarked for our dinner tables?"*

Generally, cultural traditions and food manufacturers decide this, yet there are obvious contradictions with respect to these decisions. For example, why is hay not considered a vegetable and offered on the market, but cowpeas (commonly called Black-eyed peas) are? Both foods are fed to cattle, yet people consume the cowpea but not hay. *Why is this?* Does the physical appeal of food influence our decisions to eat certain vegetation, while rejecting other vegetation? Apparently, it does.

On the other hand, most people would not eat wood or the bark of trees. These things, obviously, are not foods for humans. Although bark is vegetation, it is not appealing to our appetites. Its chemical composition makes it difficult to chew and digest. Yet, might we, through consuming nuts, certain beans and plants, be eating foods with chemical properties similar to bark? And, if cooking these things makes them edible, then cooking bark should make it edible. *But does it? Does something that is chewable make it digestible and fit for our consumption?*

Biochemical studies confirm that the chewability of something does not necessarily make it suitable for human consumption. Chewability is related to the action of our teeth and not our digestive enzymes. Something that is chewable is not necessarily safe to eat. This, too, was pointed out in previous chapters.

When health researchers point out the wrong foods, vegetables—namely beans, peas, and nuts—are not included in that group. Health researchers merely point to high fat, processed foods. For example, the American Heart Association's dietary advice states that one should *"limit foods high in saturated fat and cholesterol; and substitute it with unsaturated fat from vegetables, fish, legumes, and nuts."* The Association assumes that all vegetables or vegetation is safe to eat, including nuts.

However, are not wrong foods also foods that are biochemically designed for creatures other than humans? Are not wrong foods, vegetation that contain potent, highly toxic proteins, lipids, and carbohydrates? How many health researchers consider this aspect, particularly when vegetables are heavily recommended for consumption?

There is a dire need to distinguish the foodstuffs that are fit for humans from those fit for animals. As noted, such a distinction has been made. The Honorable Elijah Muhammad has brought this distinction to the forefront through His books, How To Eat To Live (Volumes 1 & 2). In these books, foodstuffs are distinguished according to the animals they are meant to serve. Humans are advised to avoid eating foods that are fit for other creatures.

This guidance, although unusual, is supported by research that demonstrates the biochemical interactions between the human digestive system and certain vegetation, specifically, those foods that we are accustomed to consuming. The Honorable Elijah Muhammad's position, with respect to food distinctions, is based upon the anatomical differences among various animals. The differences in digestive systems among animals denote differences among foodstuffs that serve each living creature. The digestibility of any food is based, principally, on this distinction. This was proven throughout this book.

The urgency to promote the food distinctions established in the books, How To Eat To Live bears heavily upon all. It is central to the quest to adopt dietary recommendations that ensure good health. *Does this statement imply that current dietary recommendations are inadequate?* Yes, it does, because even those who make dietary recommendations are in need of better health and longevity. As it stands, nutritionists, medical practitioners, and other health professionals confront disease and early mortality, just as those whom they advise. This fact erases any notion of a monopoly on medical and nutritional advice, regardless of the person or institution rendering this advice. Everyone is in need of a greater education about diet.

Read How To Eat To Live, Volumes 1 and 2.

Glossary

Absorption	Process by which the products of digestion pass through the alimentary tube mucosa into the blood or lymphatic system.
Acinar	Pertaining to a cell with a small sac-like dilatation: can be found in various glands.
Adenomatous	A small, circumscribed, benign tumor composed of small glandlike spaces.
Adipose	A tissue cell specialized for the synthesis and storage of fat. Such cells are bloated with globules of triglycerides, the nucleus being displaced to one side and the cytoplasm seen as a thin line around the fat droplet.
Adrenal Glands	Hormone producing glands located superior to the kidneys; each consists of medulla and cortex areas.
Adulterate	The process of making something less pure by adding inferior or unsuitable elements or substances to it.
Afferent	Carrying to or toward a center.
Agglutination	The process of grouping, clumping, or massing separate elements or objects.
Allergens	An antigen (substance that elicits an antibody response) is responsible for producing allergic reactions by inducing IgE formation. IgE antibodies, bound to basophils in circulation and mast cells in tissue, cause these cells to release chemicals when they come into contact with an allergen. These chemicals can cause injury to surrounding tissue - the visible signs of an allergy. An allergen can be almost anything which acts as an antigen to stimulate such an immune response.
Amenorrhea	Absence of menstruation, i.e. either lack of menarche or cessation of menses.
Amino Acid	Organic compound containing nitrogen, carbon, hydrogen, and oxygen; building block of protein.
Anabolism	Energy-requiring building phase of metabolism in which simpler substances are combined to form more complex substances.
Anaphylaxis	A type of immediate hypersensitivity that is triggered when allergen molecules crosslink to IgE antibodies attached to mast cells or basophils causing the release of inflammatory substances.
Anemia	Reduced oxygen-carrying ability of blood resulting from too few erythrocytes or abnormal hemoglobin.
Antibody	A protein molecule that is released by a plasma cell (a daughter cell of an antigen); an immunoglobulin.

Anticarcinogen	A substance that prevents cancer or combats cancer-causing agents.
Antinutrient	A food component that does not contribute to nutrition and may serve as a poison.
Atrophy	Reduction in size or wasting away of an organ or cell resulting from disease or lack of use.
Autonomic nervous system	Portion of the nervous system concerned with the regulation of activity of the cardiac muscle, smooth muscle, and glands.
B Cells	Lymphocytes that oversee humoral immunity; their descendents differentiate into antibody-producing plasma cells. Also called B lymphocytes.
Bile	Greenish-yellow or brownish fluid produced in and secreted by the liver, stored in the gallbladder, and released into the small intestine to emulsify fats.
Bioavailability	The degree to which a drug or other substance can be absorbed and utilized by those parts of the body on which it is intended to have an effect.
Bone Remodeling	Process involving bone formation and destruction in response to hormone and mechanical factors.
Calcitonin	Hormone released by the thyroid that promotes a decrease in the calcium levels of the blood; also called thyrocalcitonin.
Calorie (cal.)	Amount of energy needed to raise the temperature of 1 gram of water 1 Celsius. Energy exchanges associated with biochemical reactions are usually reported in kilocalories (1kcal = 1000cal) or large calories (Cal).
Cancer	A malignant, invasive cellular neoplasm that has the capability of spreading throughout the body or the body parts.
Carbohydrate	Organic compound composed of carbon, hydrogen, and oxygen; includes starches, sugars, cellulose.
Carcinogen	A substance or agent that can cause cancer. Radiation and some chemicals and viruses are carcinogens.
Cardiovascular System	Organ system which distributes the blood to deliver nutrients and removes wastes.
Catabolism	Process in which living cells break down substances into simpler substances.
Cell	The unit of structure and function in living organisms; the smallest unit capable of carrying out all the basic functions of life.
Cholecytokinin (CCK)	An intestinal hormone that stimulates gallbladder contraction and pancreatic juice release.
Cholesterol	Steroid found in animal fats as well as in most body tissue, made by the liver.
Chyme	Semifluid, creamy mass consisting of partially digested food and gastric juice.

Cloaca	Enlarged posterior end of the digestive tract of some animals. The cloaca, from the Latin word for *sewer*, is a single chamber into which pass solid and liquid waste materials.
Consensus	General or widespread agreement among all the members of a group.
Cysts	A closed sac or capsule, usually filled with fluid or semisolid material.
Degeneration	A disease process that causes a gradual deterioration in the structure of a body part with a consequent loss of the ability to function.
Denature	Changed structure of a protein resulting from the rupture of hydrogen bonds subjected to stress such as heating or enzymatic action.
Duodenum	The first or proximal portion of the small intestine, extending from the pylorus to the jejunum, so called because it is about 12 finger breadths in length.
Emulsification (emulsify)	The process of mixing lipid with water, usually through addition of an emulsifier, a compound that attracts both water and fat and prevents the mixture from separating.
Endocrine	Relating to glands that secrete hormones internally directly into the lymph or bloodstream.
Endogenous	Originating or growing within an organism or tissue.
Enzymes	Protein molecule that catalyzes chemical reactions of other substances without itself being destroyed or altered upon completion of the reaction.
Epidemic	Affecting at the same time a large number of persons in a locality, as a contagious disease.
Esophagus	A muscular tube through which food passes from the pharynx to the stomach.
Exocrine	Used to describe or relating to glands such as sweat glands or salivary glands that release a secretion through a duct to the surface of an organ.
Fatty acids	Any straight-chain single carboxyl group acid, especially those naturally occurring in fats, generally classified as saturated when they have one double bond; monounsaturated when they have one double bond; and polyunsaturated when they have multiple double bonds.
Gene	Segment of a DNA molecule that contains all the information required for synthesis of a product, biological unit of heredity.
Genitourinary	Relating to or affecting the genital and urinary organs.
Glucogen	Chief carbohydrate storage material in animals, a long-chain polymer of glucose.

Histamine	A hormone/chemical transmitter (biogenic monoamine, similar to serotonin, epinephrine, norepinephrine) involved in local immune responses, regulating stomach acid production and in allergic reactions as a mediator of Immediate Hypersensitivity.
Hypertension	Abnormally high blood pressure or arterial disease accompanied by high blood pressure.
Impermeable	Material that is not able to be penetrated or permeated.
Insoluble	Material that is incapable of being dissolved in a liquid.
Ketoacidosis	Acidosis accompanied by the accumulation of ketone bodies (ketosis) in the body tissues and fluids, as in diabetic acidosis.
Lipids	Organic compound formed of carbon, hydrogen and oxygen; examples are fats and cholesterol.
Lymphatic system	System consisting of lymphatic vessels, lymphatic nodes, and other lymphoid organs and tissues; drains excess tissue fluid from the extracelluar space and provides a site for immune surveillance.
Mast Cells	Mast cells (which are Leukocytes) contain metachromatic granules which store a variety of inflammatory mediators. These include histamine and serotonin; proteolytic enzymes that can destroy tissue or cleave complement components; heparin or chondroitin sulfate, which are anticoagulants; chemotactic factors, such as eosinophil chemotactic factor of anaphylaxis (an important regulator of eosinophil function) and neutrophil chemotactic factor. Normally, mast cells are not found in circulation.
Monogastric	Mammals with single-chambered stomachs, unlike ruminants with multi-chambered stomachs.
Monounsaturated fatty acid	A fatty acid containing one point of unsaturation.
Necrosis	The sum of the morphological changes indicative of cell death and caused by the progressive degradative action of enzymes, it may affect groups of cells or part of a structure or an organ.
Nephropathy	Pertaining to any kidney disease (e.g. nephropathy can be applied to any disease of the kidney).
Neuropathy	A general term denoting functional disturbances and/or pathological changes in the peripheral nervous system. If the involvement is in one nerve it is called mononeuropathy, in several nerves, mononeuropathy multiplex, if diffuse and bilateral, polyneuropathy.
Neurotransmitter	Any of a group of substrates that are released on excitation from the axon terminal of a presynaptic neuron of the central nervous system and travel across the synaptic cleft to either excite or inhibit the target cells.
Nodules	A small solid collection of tissue, a nodule is palpable (can be felt). It may range in size from greater than 0.5cm (3/16 inch).

Nostrum	A remedy for a social, political, or economic problem, especially an idea or scheme that is often suggested but never proved to be successful.
Obesity	Body weight of 20% or more above the appropriate weight for height.
Oxidation	The process whereby fatty acids are degraded in steps, losing 2 carbons as (acetyl) CoA. Involves CoA ester formation, desaturation, hydroxylation and oxidation before each cleavage.
Peristaltic	Progressive, wavelike contractions that move foodstuff through the alimentary tube organs (or that move other substances through other hollow body organs).
Polyunsaturated fatty acid	A fatty acid in which two or more points of unsaturation occur. The point of unsaturation is the site in a molecule where the binding is such that additional hydrogen atoms can easily be added.
Protein	Complex nitrogenous substance; main building material of cells.
Proteolysis	Splitting of proteins by hydrolysis of the peptide bonds with formation of smaller polypeptides.
Quackery	Derived from the word quacksalver (someone who boasts about his salves), a quack is a pretender to medical skill; a charlatan and one who talks pretentiously without sound knowledge of the subject discussed.
Retinopathy	Retinopathy is damage to the retina caused by microvascular changes. Microvascular disease (involving small blood vessels) due to diabetes affects the eyes and kidneys.
Saturated (fats) fatty acid	A fatty acid carrying the maximum possible number of hydrogen atoms (having no points of unsaturation), A saturated fat is a triglyceride that contains three saturated fatty acids.
Sclerosis	A induration or hardening, especially hardening of a part from inflammation and in diseases of the interstitial substance. The term is used chiefly for such a hardening of the nervous system due to hyperplasia of the connective tissue or to designate hardening of the blood vessels.
T-Cells	Lymphocytes that mediate cellular immunity; include killer, suppressor, and memory cells. Also called T-lymphocytes.
Thromboembolism	The blocking of a blood vessel by a particle that has broken away from a blood clot at its site of formation.
Triglyceride	Fats and oils composed of fatty acids and glycerol; are the body's most concentrated source of energy fuel; also known as neutral fats.
Unsaturated fatty acid	A fatty acid that lacks some hydrogen atoms and has one or more points of unsaturation. An unsaturated fat is a triglyceride that contains one or more unsaturated fatty acid.

Bibliography

1. Association AD. Americans' Food and Nutrition Attitudes and Behaviors. Chicago: American Dietetic Association, 2000.
2. Klurfeld DM, Kritchevsky D. The Western diet: An examination of its relationship with chronic disease. Journal of American College of Nutrition 1986;5(5):477-85.
3. Weisburger JH. Dietary fat and risk of chronic disease: mechanistic insights from experimental studies. Journal of American Dietetic Association 1997;Supplement 7:S16-23.
4. National Health Expenditures, 1998. Baltimore: Health Care Financing Administration, 2000;www.hcfa.gov.
5. Kong D. Milk as a Food Requirement Is Questioned. Vol. 99 PR Newswire, 1999.
6. Organization WH. Conquering Suffering: Enriching Humanity. Geneva: World Health Organization, 1997.
7. Ory RL, Flick GJ. Peanuts. In: Macrae R, Robinson RK, Sadler MJ, eds. Encyclopedia of Food Science, Food Technology, and Nutrition. Vol. 5. New York: Academic Press, 1993;3473-3477.
8. Association AD. Health Snacking--Nuts To You. Tip of the Day 1996.
9. Prevention NCfCDPaHPCD. The Burden of Cardiovascular Diseases,Cancer, and Diabetes. Washing: Centers for Disease Control and Prevention, 1999.
10. Kulman L. While diet docs debate fats and carbs, weight loss still comes down to calories. U.S. News & World Report, 2000.
11. Committee DGA. Report of the Dietary Guidelines Advisory Committee on the Dietary Guidelines for Americans, 2000. Washington, D.C.: United States Department of Agriculture, 2000;187.
12. Willett WC. What should we eat? Science 1994;264:532-537.
13. Pearson' TA, Kirwan JP, Maddox D, Fishell V, Juturu V, Kris-Etherton PM. Weight loss and Weight Maintenance: Effects of High MUFA vs Low Fat Diets on Plasma Lipids and Lipoproteins. Experimental Biology 1999;Presentation(April 19).
14. Abbey M, Noakes M, Belling G, Nestel P. Partial Replacement of Saturated Fatty Acids with Almonds or Walnuts Lowers Total Plasma Cholesterol and Low-Density-Lipoprotein Cholesterol. American Journal of Clinical Nutrition 1994;59:995-9.
15. Curb JD, Wergowske G, Dobbs J, Abbott RD, Huang B. Comparison of Lipid Levels in Humans on a Macadamia Nut Based High Monounsaturated Fat Diet and a High Fat Typical American Diet. Presentation, American Heart Association, Scientific Conference on Efficacy of Hypocholesterolemic Dietary Interventions 1995:3-5.

16. Sabate J, Fraser GE, Burke K, Knutsen SF, Bennett H, Lindsted KD. Effects of Walnuts on Serum Lipid Levels and Blood Pressure in Normal Men. The New England Journal of Medicine 1993;328(9).

17. Dreher ML, Maher C, Kearney P. The Traditional and Emerging Role of Nuts in Healthful Diets. Nutritional Reviews 1996;54:241-5.

18. Pearson TA, Etherton TD, Moriarty K, Reed R, Kris-Etherton PM. High-Monounsaturated Fatty Acid Diets with Peanuts-Peanut Butter or Peanut Oil Lower Total Cholesterol and LDL-C Identically to a Step 2 Diet But Eliminate the Triglyceride Increase. Experimental Biology 1998;Presentation(April 20).

19. Lermer CM, Mattes RM. Effects of Chronic Peanut Consumption on Body Weight and Serum Lipid Levels in Humans. Presentation 1999(April 19).

20. Mattes RD, Voisard SK. Effects of Peanuts on Hunger and Food Intakes in Humans. Experimental Biology 1998;Presentation(April 20).

21. Fraser G, Sabate J, Beeson LW, Strahan MT. A Possible Effect of Nut Consumption on Risk of Coronary Heart Disease. Archives of Internal Medicine 1992;152:1416-24.

22. O'Byrne DJ, Knauff DA, Shireman RB. Low-Fat Monounsaturated Rich Diets Containing High-Oleic Peanut Improve Serum Lipoprotein Profiles. Lipids 1997;32:687-95.

23. Eissenstat B, Juturu V, Hshieh G, Maddox D, Kris-Etherton PM. Impact of Consuming Peanuts and Peanut Products on Energy and Nutrient Intakes of American Adults. Experimental Biology 1999;Presentation(April 19).

24. Brown L, Rosner BA, Willet WC, Sacks FM. Nut Consumption and Risk of Recurrent Coronary Heart Disease. Experimental Biology 1999;Presentation(April 19).

25. Wanda A. Morgan P, RD, Beverly J. Clayshulte M. Pecans lower-density lipoprotein cholesterol. Journal of the American Dietetic Association 2000;100:312-318.

26. Hu FB, Stampfer MJ, Manson JE, Colditz GA, Rosner BA, Speizer FE, Hennekens CH, Willett WC. Frequent nut consumption and risk of coronary heart disease in women: prospective cohort study. British Medical Journal 1998;317:1341-1345.

27. Prineas RJ, Kushi LH, Folsom AR, Bostick RM. Letter to the Editor. New England Journal of Medicine 1993;329:359.

28. Albert CM, Willet WC, Manson JE, Hennekens CH. Nut Consumption and the Risk of Sudden and Total Cardiac Death in the Physicians Health Study. American Heart Association 1998;Abstract(November 9-11).

29. Award AB, Chan K, Downie A, Fink CS. Anticancer Properties. Experimental Biology 1999;Presenation(April 19).

30. Young JH. The Medical Messiahs. Princeton, New Jersey: Princeton University Press, 1967.

31. Backgrounder F. Milestones in U.S. Food and Drug Law History. Washington, D.C.: Federal Food and Drug Administration, 1999.

32. Young JH. American Health Quackery. New Jersey: Princeton University Press, 1992.

33. Marsa L. Prescription for Profits. New York, NY: Scribner, 1997.

34. FDA. Rezulin to be withdrawn from the market. HHS News. Washington, D.C.:, 2000.

35. Press TA. Fen-Phen Articles Questioned "Drug Maker Accused of Funding Favorable Journal Articles". Vol. 1999 ABC News Website (abcnews.com), 1999.

36. Ensminger AH, Ensminger ME, Konlande JE, Robson JRK. Legumes. In: Ensminger AH, ed. The Concise Encyclopedia of Food & Nutrition. Boca Raton, FL: CRC Press, 1995;608.

37. Koch T. Splanchnology. In: Skold BH, ed. Anatomy of the Chicken and Domestic Birds. Ames, Iowa: The Iowa State University Press, 1973;66-90.

38. Vaidehi MP, Kadam SS. Peanut. In: Salunkhe DK, ed. CRC Handbook of World Food Legumes. Vol. 2. Baca Raton, FL: CRC Press, 1990;198.

39. Liener IE, Kakade ML. Protease Inhibitors. In: Liener IE, ed. Toxic Constituents of Plant Foodstuffs. 2nd. ed. New York: Academic Press, 1980.

40. Birk Y, Gertler A. Chemistry and biology of proteinase inhibitors from soybeans and groundnuts. International Research Conference on Proteinase Inhibitors: W. De Gruyter, 1970.

41. Lotan R, Skutelsky E, Canon D, Sharon N. The purification, composition and specificity of the anti-T lectin from peanuts. Journal of Biological Chemistry 1975;250:8518.

42. Miller RL. Purification of peanut (Arachis hypogaea) agglutinin isolectins by chromatofocusing. Analytical Biochemistry 1983;131:438.

43. Sitren HS, Ahmed EM, George DE. In vivo and in vitro assessment of antinutritional factors in peanut and soy. Journal of Food Science 1985;58:418.

44. Cheryan M. Phytic acid interactions in food systems. CRC Critical Reviews of Food Science and Nutrition, 1980.

45. Maga JA. Phytate: its chemistry, occurence, food interactions, nutritional significance, and methods of analysis. Journal of Agriculture Food Chemistry 1982;30:1.

46. Reddy NR, Sathe SK, Salunke DK. Phytates in legumes ad cereals. Advances and Food Research 1982;28:1.

47. Macfarlane BJ, Bezwoda WR, Bothwell TH, Baynes RD, Bothwell JE, MacPhail A, Lamparelli RD, Mayet F. Inhibitory effect of nuts on iron absorption. American Journal of Clinical Nutrition 1988;47:270-274.

48. Gillooly M, Bothwell TH, Torrance JD. The effects of organic acids, phytates and polyphenols on the absorption of iron from vegetables. British Journal of Nutrition 1983;49:331-41.

49. Vaintraub IA, Bulmaga VP. Effects of phytate on the in vitro activity of digestive enzymes. Journal of Agriculture Food Chemistry 1991;39:859.

50. Singh M, Krikorian AD. Inhibition of trypsin activity in vitro by phytate. Journal of Agriculture Food Chemistry 1982;30:799.

51. Caldwell RA. Effect of calcium and phytate acid on the activation of trypsinogen and the stability of trypsin. Journal of Agriculture Food Chemistry 1992;40:43.

52. Sharma CB, Goel M, Irshad M. Myoinositol hexaphosphate as a potential inhibitor of amylases. Phytochemistry 1978;17:2101.

53. Deshpande SS, Cheryan M. Effects of phytic acid, divalent cations, and their interaction on amylase activity. Journal of Food Science 1984;49:516.

54. Knuckles BE, Betschart AA. Effect of phytate and other myo-inositol phosphate esters on amylase digestion of starch. Journal of Food Science 1987;52:719.

55. Knuckles BE, Kuzmicky DD, Betschart AA. Effect of phytate and partially hydrolyzed phytate on in vitro protein digestibility. Journal of Food Science 1985;50:1080.

56. Greer MA, Asherwood EB. The antithyroid effect of certain foods in man as determined with radioactive iodine. Endocrinology 1948;43:105.

57. Prevention CfDCa. About Chronic Disease: Definition, Overall Burden, and Cost Effectiveness of Prevention. Washington, D.C.: U.S. Department of Health & Human Services, 1998;2.

58. Ham WW, Sandstedt RM, Mussehl FE. The proteolytic inhibiting substance in the extract from unheated soybean meal and its effect upon growth. Journal of Biological Chemistry 1945;161:635.

59. Kakade ML, Hoffa DE, Leiner IE. Contribution of trypsin inhibitors to the deleterious effects of unheated soybeans fed to rats. Journal of Nutrition 1973;103:1172.

60. Chernick SS, Lepkovsky S, Chaikoff IL. A dietary factor regulating the enzyme content of the pancreas; changes induced in the size and the proteolytic activity of the chick pancreas by the ingestion of raw soybean meal. American Journal of Physiology 1948;155:33.

61. Lyman RL, Wilcox SA, Monsen ER. Pancreatic enzyme secretion produced in the rat by trypsin and chymotrypsin inhibitors. American Journal of Physiology 1962;202:1077.

62. Hathcock JN, Center for Food Safety and Applied Nutrition FaDA. Residue trypsin inhibitor: data needs for risk assessment. Advancements in Experimental Medical Biology 1991;289:273-9.

63. Lyman RL, Lepkovsky S. The effect of raw soybean meal and trypsin inhibitor diets on pancreatic enzyme secretion in the rat. Journal of Nutrition 1957;62:269.

64. Booth AN, Robbins DJ, Ribelin WE, De Eds F. Effects of raw soybean meal and amino acids on pancreatic hypertrophy in rats. Proceedings of Society of Experimental Biological Medicine 1960;104:681.

65. Levison DA, Morgan RG, Brinacomb JS, Hopwood D, Coghill G, Wormsley KG. Carcinogenic effects of di(hydroxypropoly) nitrosamine (DHPN) in male Wistar rats: promotion of pancreatic cancer by raw soya flour diet. Scandanavian Journal of Gastroenterology 1979;14:217.

66. J. W. Erdman J. Soy products and the human diet. American Journal of Clinical Nutrition 1989;49(5):728.

67. Holm H, Hanssen LE, Krogdahl A, Floholmen J. High and Low Inhibitor Soybean Meals Affect Human Doudenal Proteinase Activity Differently: In Vivo Comparison with Bovine Serum Albumin. Journal of Nutrition 1988;118:515-520.

68. Mellitus ECotDaCoD. Report of the Expert Committee on the Diagnosis and Classification of Diabetes Mellitus. Diabetes Care 2000;23(Supplement):S4-S19.

69. Sundqvist T, Lindstrom F, Magnusson K, Skoldstam L, Stjernstrom I, Tagesson C. Influence of Fasting on Intestinal Permeability and Disease Activity in Patients with Rheumatoid Arthritis. Scandanavian Journal of Rheumatology 1982;11:33-38.

70. Kjeldsen-Kragh JH, M; Haugen, M; Forre, O. Antibodies against dietary antigens in rheumatoid arthritis patients treated with fasting and a one-year-vegatarian diet. Clinical and Experimental Rheumatology 1995;13(2):167.

71. Peltonen RK-K, J.; Haugen, M; Tuominen, J. Changes of faecal flora in rheumatoid arthritis during fasting and one-year vegetarian diet. British Journal of Rheumatolgy 1994;33(7):638.

72. Prevention CfDCa. Diabetes: A Serious Public Health Problem At-A-Glance 2000. Washington, D.C.: U.S. Department of Health and Human Services, 2000.

73. Promotion NCfCDPaH. Chronic Diseases and Condition: Arthritis. Vol. 2000 Centers for Disease Control and Prevention.

74. Joseph g. Hollowell NWS, W. Harry Hannon, Dana W. Flanders, et al. Iodine Nutrition in the United States. Trends and Public Health Implications: Iodine Excretion Data from National Health and Nutrition Examination Surveys I and III (1971-1974 and 1988-1994). Journal of Clinical Endocrinology and Metabolism 1998;83(10):34013407.

75. womenshealth.about.com. Depression and Women. Vol. 2000 Women's Health, 2000.

76. Bleichrodt N, Born MP. A metaanalysis of research on iodine and its relationship to cognitive development. In: Stanbury JB, ed. The damaged brain of iodine deficiency: cognitive, behavioral, neuromotor, and educative aspects. New York: Cognizant Communication Corp, 1994;195-200.

77. Tiwari BD, Godbole MM, Chattopadhyay N, Mandel A, Mithal A. Learning disabilities and poor motivation to achieve due to prolonged iodine deficiency. American Journal Clinical Nutrition 1996;63:782-786.

78. Kimball OP. Endemic goiter-a food deficiency disease. Journal of American Dietetic Association 1949;25:112-115.

79. Pennington JAT, Schoen SA. Contributions of food groups to estimated intakes of nutritional elements: results from the FDA Total Diet Studies 1982-1991. International Journal for Vitamin and Nutrition Research 1996;66:350-362.

80. Staff. The thyroid: your "get-up-and-go" gland. University of Texas Lifetime Health Letter 1997;8(August 9):4-6.

81. Underwood A. It's All In Your Neck. Newsweek, 1998;63-64.

82. Gay J. Canaris M, MSPH, Neil R. Manowitz P, Gilbert Mayor M, E. Chester Ridgway M. The Colorado Thyroid Disease Prevalence Study. Archives of Internal Medicine 2000;160(4):526-534.

83. Morgan P. Unmasking Thyroid Trouble. Prevention 1997;91:162-164, 166.

84. Promotion CfNPa, Agriculture USDo. Childhood Obesity:Causes & Prevention Symposium Proceedings. Washington, D.C., 1998.

85. Kuczmarski RJ, Flegal KM, Campbell SM, Johnson CL. Increasing prevalence of overweight among U.S. adults. The National Health and Nutrition Examination Surveys. JAMA 1994;272:205-211.

86. Astrup A, Buemann B, Toubro S, Ranneries C, Raben A. Low resting metabolic rate in subjects predisposed to obesity: a role for thyroid status. American Journal of Clinical Nutrition 1996;63:879-83.

87. Weinberg RA. How Cancer Arises. Scientific American, 1996;62-70.

88. PRNewswire. Americans Urged to 'Take Cholesterol by the Neck'. PRNewswire. New York:, 2000;2.

89. Gibbons GF, Mitropoulos KA, Bryant NB. Biochemistry of Cholesterol. Amsterdam: Elsevier, 1982.

90. Michael D. Gershon MD. The Second Brain. New York, NY: Harper Collins Publishers, 1998.

91. Mohammad Masud Iqbal M, MPH, MSPH. Osteoporosis: Epidemiology, Diagnosis, and Treatment. Southern Medical Journal 2000;93(1):2-18.

92. Manolagas S. Combination of Estrogen and Parathyroid Hormone Injections Produce Dramatic Increases in Bone Density in Postmenopausal Osteoporosis. Advances in the Treatment of Osteoporosis. St. Louis, MO: Medscape Diabetes & Endocrinology, 1999.

93. Manolagas S. Low and Intermittent Doses of Parathyroid Hormone Promote Bone Formation. Advances in the Treatment of Osteoporosis. St. Louis, MO: Medscape Diabetes & Endocrinology, 1999.

94. Kothari, Shakuntala, Thacker, Holly L. Risk assessment of the menopausal patient. The Medical Clinics of North America 1999;83(6):1489.

95. Tish Lafferty R, MSN. Hormone Replacement Choices for Women in Midlife. Vol. 2000 Meriter Women's Health Online, Meriter Women and Family Center, 1999.

96. Progestin adds to breast cancer risk. Science News 2000(March 11).

97. Grady D, Wenger NK, Herrington D, Khan S, Furberg C, Hunninghake D, Vittinghoff E, Hulley S. Postmenopausal Hormone Therapy Increases Risk for Venous Thromboembolic Disease. The Heart and Estrogen/progestin Replacement Study. Annuals of Internal Medicine 2000;132(9):689-696.

98. Beatriz R. Olson MD. Teaching Rounds: Facets of Thyroid Disease in Women: Four Case Reports. Women's Health 1998;7(1):85-92.

99. Dratman MB. Thyroid Hormones as neurotransmitters. Thyroid 1996;6:639-47.

100. Bothwell TH, Charlton RW, Cook JD, Finch CA. Iron metabolism in man. Blackwell Scientific Publications. Oxford:, 1979.

101. Eigenmann PA, Sampson HA. Adverse Reactions to Foods. In: Allen P. Kaplan M, ed. Allergy. 2nd ed. Stony Brook, NY: W.B. Saunders Company;542-560.

102. Bargman TJ, Rupnow JH, Taylor SL. IgE-binding proteins in almonds (Prunus amygdalus) identified by immunoblotting with sera from almond-allergic adults. Journal of Food Science 1992;57(3):717-20.

103. Arshad SH, Malamberg E, Krapf K, Hide DW. Clinical and immunological characteristics of Brazil nut allergy. Clinical and Experimental Allergy 1991;21:373-76.

104. Wickens GE. Edible Nut. FAO Rome 1995.

105. Bush RK, Hefle SL. Food Allergens. Critical Reviews in Food Science and Nutrition 1996;36S:S119-63.

106. Falliers CJ. Pine nut allergy in perspective. Annals of Allergy 1989;62:186-89.

107. Sampson HA, Medelson L, Rosen JP. Fatal and near-fatal anaphylactic reactions to food in children and adolescent. New England Journal of Medicine 1992;327(6):380-84.

108. Anon. Nut allergy kills woman at party. Daily Telegraph, 1996.

109. Hide D. Clinical curio: allergy to Brazil nut. British Medical Journal 1993;287:900.

110. Marks JG, DeMelfi T, McCarthy MA, Witte EJ, Castagnoli N, Epstein WI, Aber RC. Dermatitis from cashew nuts. Journal of the American Academy of Dermatology 1984;10(4):627-31.

111. Parra FM, Cuevas M, Lezaun A. Pistachio nut hypersensitivity: identification of pistachio nut allergens. Clinical and Experimental Allergy 1993;23:996.

112. Yunginger JW, Sweeney KG, Sturner WQ. Fatal food-induced anaphylaxis. Journal of the American Medical Association 1988;260(10):1450-52.

113.Fine AJ. Hypersensitivity reaction to pine nuts (pinon nuts--Pignolia). Annals of Allergy 1987;48:220-226.

114.Golbert TM, Patterson R, Pruzansky JJ. Systemic allergic reactions to ingested antigens. Journal of Allergy 1969;32:96-107.

115.Clark S. Problem peanuts: Peanut allergy is increasing and those at risk of anaphylaxis must take extreme caution. Nursing Standard 1996;10(38):25.

116.Frank L, Marian A, Visser M, Weinberg E, Potter PC. Exposure to peanuts in utero and in infancy and the development of sensitization to peanut allergens in young children. Pediatric Allergy and Immunology 1999;10(1):27.

117.Chrandra RK. Food hypersensitivity and allergic disease: a selective review. American Journal of Clinical Nutrition 1997;66:526S-529S.

118.Section H. Banning Peanuts. Newsweek. Vol. 132, 1998;77.

119.L. Life-Threatening Allergies Spur Peanut Bans at Mass. Schools. Education Week 1996.

120.Eigenmann M, A. Wesley Burks M, Gary A. Bannon P, Hugh A. Sampson M. Identification of unique peanut and soy allergens in sera absorbed with cross-reacting antibodies. Journal of Allergy and Clinical Immunology 1996;98(5).

121.Christiansen SC, Zuraw BL. Allergy. In: Dulbecco R, ed. Encyclopedia of Human Biology. Vol. 1. La Jolla, CA: Academic Press, 1997;249-262.

122.Promotional Insights. www.scottlevin.com: Scott Levin Online, 2000.

123.Dietz J. U.S. Doctors Average 2,060 Prescriptions in '99. www.scottlevin.com. Newtown, PA:, 2000.

124.Denise. Synthroid/Thyroid Problems!!?? Please Read. In: Members HMB, ed. www.homefirst.com/wwwboard/messages/1655.html: Homefirst Message Board, 1999.

125. S. Jay Olshanky BAC, and Christine K. Cassel. In Search of Methuselah: Estimating the Upper Limits to Human Longevity. Science 1990;250(November 2):634-40.

Index

Z